Book Description

Are you a woman over 50? Do you want to take control of your body, increase your vitality, and lose weight?

Are you tired of the gimmicky fad diets that rear their heads at every turn without proof or scientific data behind their claims? Are you looking for a weight loss or health regime that works with your body's natural processes?

If you are a woman over 50, you are likely experiencing all of the changes that this new phase of life brings to us—most of these are positive, but some are a little challenging. We should be celebrating this stage of our lives and not desperately trying to wade through the murky waters of menopausal uncertainty.

That's where intermittent fasting comes in.

Intermittent fasting is an ancient practice that has been revived for modern times. It is one of the few health and weight loss regimes for which there is not only a large amount of scientific backing but also an incredible number of personal testimonies to support its efficacy.

In ***Intermittent Fasting For Women Over 50***, we teach you the principles of intermittent fasting and focus them directly on your very specific needs as a woman over 50.

Weight gain is one of the side-effects of aging that we as women have come to see as unavoidable, especially when it comes to post-menopausal weight gain. Thankfully, weight gain at this time in your life is not only completely avoidable, but it is also really quite easy to achieve.

Your body is actually designed to work with the principles of fasting to increase your vitality and longevity and help fight disease. All you have to do is learn how to activate those pre-programmed processes.

In *Intermittent Fasting For Women Over 50*, you will learn how to:

- **Activate your body's processes through fasting**
- Decrease the impact that menopause has on your life and health
- Make intermittent fasting a flexible and enjoyable part of your lifestyle

- Choose the right intermittent fasting method for you
- **Lose weight and keep it off, even during menopause**

Those are just a few points that we will cover in *Intermittent Fasting For Women Over 50*. The book is designed in such a way that when you reach the final page, your path ahead will be absolutely clear, and you will be able to immediately start enjoying the benefits that fasting can bring to your life.

In addition, we have also included detailed recipes with nutritional information to help you bring fasting principles into your kitchen, and we have provided you with our tried-and-tested recommendations for specific foods to break your fast and to keep you feeling full for longer.

As a woman over 50, you deserve to start enjoying your life and empowering yourself now. Intermittent fasting is the ideal way to minimize the challenges associated with menopause, reduce the likelihood that you will develop a serious disease, and increase your energy levels.

If you are ready to successfully conquer this new phase of your life, this book is your most valuable resource!

Intermittent Fasting For Women Over 50

A Complete Guide on Intermittent Fasting Techniques Suitable for Women Over 50

Ana M. Hil

acknowledge that the author is not engaged in the rendering of legal, financial, medical or professional advice. The content within this book has been derived from various sources. Please consult a licensed professional before attempting any techniques outlined in this book.

By reading this document, the reader agrees that under no circumstances is the author responsible for any losses, direct or indirect, that are incurred as a result of the use of the information contained within this document, including, but not limited to, errors, omissions, or inaccuracies.

Table of Contents

Introduction

Women over 50 are the powerhouses of the world. From an emotional perspective, we are no longer as easily impacted by the negativity of the world as we were in our 20s, for instance. We have embraced our strong, feisty, and fierce personalities, and we no longer feel the need to apologize for our fantastic femininity. We have helped our families grow and supported our partners through their own goals and ambitions. We are at a time in our lives when we are celebrating exactly who we are, and we have also learned the value of taking care of our bodies.

Most women over 50 have likely engaged in some form of diet in their lifetimes and are probably in a place where they are able to acknowledge that fad diets do more harm than good to their bodies in the long-run. As we age, our body chemistry changes, our energy needs are different, and we need to adapt to these changes in order to maintain a healthy weight and ensure that we protect our bodies from illness. The reason that fad diets are never a good idea is that there is so little research done into the long-term effects of such diets. No one really knows what happens in a body over 20 or 30 years when certain food groups are restricted and diets are strictly manipulated. The key to managing our weight, increasing our vitality, and protecting our health is, therefore, relying on a tried-and-tested method that has been used for centuries to improve health.

The concept of fasting is age-old. It is referred to in some of the most ancient texts in history, and even the earliest healers understood and recorded its benefits for the human body. Many cultures and religions have held onto the practice of fasting, and even today, special religious days are marked by fasting.

The Westernized world, however, has allowed itself to become overwhelmed with the instant access to food that we now have. We have a supermarket on every corner, takeout food at our beck-and-call, and instant foods that we just pop in a microwave. We don't even need to leave the house anymore to get access to food with supermarkets and takeout services delivering at the drop of a hat. As a result, we overeat, and we have convinced ourselves that the healthiest way of eating is when we eat throughout the day.

Myths and legends about eating have been drummed into our heads since we were children. "Three square meals a day" was where it started, then we were told that actually, it's healthier to split that into six smaller meals, and of course, there is the constant refrain of "breakfast is the most important meal of the day." We have become a society of constant snackers thinking that the more often we eat, the quicker our body will work to burn off the calories. We have lost the value that fasting provides to our health both physically and mentally. Thankfully, though, there has been a resurgence of fasting in recent years in the form of intermittent fasting, and the world has started to once again recognize its benefits.

As women over 50, we know very well that when it comes to our health, there is no 'one size fits all' option. We have very specific health concerns, and our bodies respond differently to weight loss techniques. You have likely tried several plans by now and perhaps become despondent at their inefficacy and the side effects you have experienced. *Intermittent Fasting For*

Women Over 50 has been written specifically with you in mind.

In this book, we approach intermittent fasting not as a diet or fad but as a lifestyle and one that will help you to achieve your weight loss goals without the yo-yoing that you have likely experienced with other methods. In the chapters that follow, we will explain the concept of intermittent fasting and the science that backs it up. The latter is something that is missing from the explanations of many weight loss methods, and that is usually because there is no scientific backing for those methods. This is one of the many ways that intermittent fasting is different.

One of the most attractive parts of the intermittent fasting lifestyle is that it is highly malleable to your own needs and routine, and there are several protocols to choose from. We will explain all of the available protocols in detail so that you can choose the best option for you. Rather than insisting that you eat a specific menu and providing some vague details about how the plan should work, we will provide you with some practical tips on how to incorporate intermittent fasting into your life and maintain it as a lifestyle going forward. While you can certainly just use intermittent fasting as an occasional tool for weight loss, in order to experience all of the benefits, we highly recommend deciding to do this as a permanent part of your life.

The flexibility of intermittent fasting revolves around the multitude of protocols available, ranging from the shortest 16:8 protocol to longer, extended fasts. By using these different protocols, you can bend the lifestyle to fit what is happening in your life at the time. Over the festive season, you may want to look at a 5:2 protocol, where you only fast for 2 days out of the week, but those fasts are longer. Then when you are back into your normal routine again, you can do a more regular daily pattern of fasting. In this way, no matter what is happening in your life, you never lose out on the benefits of fasting. Even during times when we would ordinarily be spending a lot of time at parties and get-togethers with friends and family and would end up feeling like the stuffed turkey we consumed, fasting will very quickly put you back in a more comfortable state.

Another way that intermittent fasting is different from other diets or eating plans is that its benefits are not just health-related.

Intermittent fasting has benefits for your mental health and emotional health as well. One of the most difficult parts of menopause is experiencing erratic mood shifts due to hormone changes that can really disrupt our lives and have us behaving in ways we ordinarily wouldn't. Fasting can help stabilize blood sugar and hormone levels so that we can get back to being who we know ourselves to be.

As with any new lifestyle, there will be some challenges in the beginning, but we will approach those with you and help you to overcome them by giving you various solutions to the challenges you may come across. Included in *Intermittent Fasting For Women Over 50* is a chapter containing some fasting-friendly food suggestions as well as simple recipes that will help you to bring intermittent fasting into your kitchen.

Aging has its health challenges, especially for women. It is entirely impossible to live a healthy, happy life while still enjoying delicious and exciting meals. Intermittent fasting is a journey that will lead to a greater feeling of vitality and wellness than you ever imagined possible. *Intermittent Fasting For Women Over 50* is your roadmap for that journey, and we look forward to guiding you and assisting you in accomplishing your ultimate health and wellness goals.

Chapter 1: What Is Intermittent Fasting?

You are likely already familiar with the term 'fasting,' perhaps having heard it in relation to religious practices or something you had to do before blood tests or an operation. It most likely creates an image in your head of draconian practices in which people punish themselves for their sins. You may think that fasting means not eating. Intermittent fasting, however, has nothing to do with starving yourself. The term 'starvation' implies that you do not have access to food and that you are, in some way, experiencing negative health effects from not eating. Starvation is generally not deliberate or controlled.

Instead, intermittent fasting means that although you do have access to food, you *choose* when to eat and the experience is not damaging to your health in the way that starvation would be. Intermittent fasting involves assigning a pattern for eating around specific times.

You may be wondering how that is any different from eating breakfast, lunch, and dinner at specific times. If you consider the fact that you usually don't eat meals at specific times but rather when and if you are hungry, that shows a distinct difference between the two ideas. When you practice intermittent fasting, you structure your day in fasting hours and eating hours. There are various time-based protocols which we will discuss later in this book through which you can attribute different time periods to fasting and eating. The essential idea, though, is that you allocate a period of the day in which you do not eat and then a period of the day in which you do eat. Intermittent fasting is different from other eating plans in that it does not determine what you can eat but rather when you should eat.

The term "intermittent fasting" was the most popular diet-related reference in search engines in 2019 with a 10,000 percent increase in the search for this term since 2010 (Fung, 2020). One of the most popular methods of intermittent fasting that we can use to illustrate the concept is the 16:8 protocol. In this protocol, you fast for 16 hours and then you have an eating window of eight hours. Considering you are already not eating while you sleep, which should ideally be for eight hours, the idea is to extend that period for another eight hours. This would, therefore, mean if you go to sleep at 10 pm and wake up at 6 am, you would then not eat until 2 pm. From 2 pm to 10 pm, you can eat a small light lunch and then your dinner at least two hours before you go to sleep for digestion purposes.

This is the basis of intermittent fasting, which, in itself, will provide you with a myriad of health benefits. If you decide that you also want to specifically lose a certain amount of weight as well, you will need to limit the number of calories you take in during your eating window and increase your activity. During your fasting window, you should take in no food, but you can drink beverages that have little to no caloric content such as water or coffee and tea with no milk or sugar. You can take supplements during your fasting period, but if possible, you may want to delay taking the supplements until your eating period since taking them on an empty stomach can make you feel nauseous.

Intermittent fasting is a very natural way of structuring our eating. Before we had a constant supply of food on demand, fasting was the norm, and it is still a very natural process for many animals, some of which don't eat for weeks or months at a time while hibernating. Our hunter-gatherer ancestors, after all, did not have the luxury of constant access to food, so fasting was not really a choice for them, but they survived some seriously difficult conditions all the same.

Our energy requirements are, of course, very different today than they were during the age that we had to hunt our own food. At that time, we needed bursts of energy in order to overcome situations that occasionally cropped up. Today, our energy requirements are more sustained, so it stands to reason that we would not fast for extended periods.

It does take a mindset change to introduce intermittent fasting as a lifestyle since you have likely grown up with the idea that having three square meals per day is the healthiest way to eat. We have also had phrases like "breakfast is the most important meal of the day" drummed into our heads, which is usually just a marketing tool for sugar-filled cereal brands.

An intermittent fasting lifestyle has a huge number of health benefits including weight loss, fat burning, stabilization of blood sugar, limiting of disease, increased rate of cell repair, and increased longevity.

In explaining what intermittent fasting is, it is perhaps pertinent to explain what it is not. Intermittent fasting is not a free ticket to binge on everything your eyes see as long as you 'starve' yourself within the required period. Anyone approaching intermittent fasting from such a standpoint is doing themselves more harm than good. The basics of good nutrition—lean proteins, plenty of fresh fruit and vegetables, good sources of fiber, and good fats—do not change because you are structuring the times at which you eat. If you wish to see all of the benefits that intermittent fasting can offer, then maintaining good nutrition with the occasional treat is imperative.

One of the downsides of the sudden burst in popularity of intermittent fasting is that there are people who will tout it as a fad diet and make recommendations around suggested protocols that are not good for your health. Educating yourself around the principles of fasting as a practice and how your body works when it is fasting is the key to not being taken in by one of these misguided trends. True intermittent fasting does not describe a condition under which you can constantly overindulge during your eating windows as long as you 'deprive' yourself during your fasting window.

Another important factor to consider in understanding intermittent fasting is the period of time for which you fast. Abstaining from food in the intermittent fasting lifestyle is never intended to be prolonged. There are protocols that dictate a 24-hour long fast, and for expert-level fasters, this is fine, but for beginners, it is not recommended. Any period longer than 24-hours is not recommended for anyone.

As we will delve into in deeper detail later, intermittent fasting is quite flexible as long as you stick to the basic ideas behind it and ensure that what you are doing is promoting health. If your goal is weight loss, it is important to understand that intermittent fasting will help you lose weight relatively quickly, but it does so in a healthy manner. If you do not continue with an intermittent fasting lifestyle after losing the weight you want to, you are at risk of gaining weight again. At the very least, you must commit to maintaining a lower caloric intake and a higher caloric burning through increased activity.

This book gives you a huge amount of information on intermittent fasting, but it is important to continuously refresh and recharge your knowledge. Do ensure that you are choosing your sources of knowledge wisely, though, and stick to reputable experts and websites. The great thing about intermittent fasting is that you will very quickly become knowledgeable on the subject just by practicing the lifestyle. As you continue on your journey, if you notice certain things happening in your body that didn't before, do some research to see what processes within the body are causing it. This is how we get to know our bodies. Even at 50, we have the capacity to learn about our bodies, and it is vital to be open to new possibilities.

Chapter 2: The Science Behind Intermittent Fasting

Most eating plans will avoid discussing the science behind their methods since, in most cases, the research is vague and contradictory. There is a significant risk in jumping from diet to diet in order to try and find something that works for you, and the unfortunate effect that this may have on your body in the future may only be known when it is too late. It is really not worth the risk. While it is important to keep your weight at a healthy level, it is equally important to do so in a manner that doesn't further damage your body. If you are looking at a particular dict in order to lose weight, be sure to do your research. One study on animal participants only does not constitute research.

By the same token, 'proof' based solely on testimonials is also not conclusive enough. After all, you don't know these people, and you have no idea whether they really lost "50 pounds in a single day on the Caramel Popcorn Diet" (In case it's not clear, there is no Caramel Popcorn Diet. If there was, we would be on it!). The diet industry is just that, an industry, and industries are there to make money. Of course, it is entirely possible to make money ethically, give people sound advice, and see them get real benefits, but the opposite is just as possible.

Thankfully, this is not the case with intermittent fasting. Not only are there hundreds of years of real-world proof of the benefits, but there is a huge amount of research in laboratories and other studies that can be relied upon. The impact of fasting on very specific areas of the body can also be measured and explained through scientific processes that medical doctors will confirm.

The brilliance of intermittent fasting is its simplicity. There are protocols and add-ons that can be built on around intermittent fasting, but the very basic scientific principles always remain. It's a tried-and-tested concept, as evidenced by references to fasting in some of the most ancient texts in history. Even today, many cultures and religions still hold on to the ancient practices of fasting because they really do bring benefits.

If you are still unsure about whether intermittent fasting is medically right for you after reading *Intermittent Fasting For Women Over 50*, you should consult a medical professional and get their take on it. Sometimes, it just takes a face-to-face qualified opinion to convince you that something is in your best interest.

But how, exactly, does fasting work?

What Happens in Your Body When You Fast?

When we eat, our body converts food into glucose. There is very limited space for the storage of glucose, though, so as soon as that limit is reached, the body will start to store the rest of the food as fat. This fat production process is called denovo lipogenesis. The capacity for storage of fat, in contrast to glucose, is unlimited, so if you continue to take in food before burning off your glucose resources, your body will continue making and storing fat (Fung, 2016). When this is happening inside our body, what we experience on the outside is that feeling of a slowly expanding waistline, your body feeling flabbier than usual, and a general decline in how you feel about yourself.

The science behind intermittent fasting starts with insulin levels. Insulin is a hormone that our pancreas produces that helps our body to turn carbohydrates into glucose. Glucose is the body's energy source and what it uses to burn as fuel to power your body's various processes. Our body releases insulin at the rate at which we take in food, so if we are not taking in food for a prolonged period, our insulin levels drop. When this happens, our body will first burn any stored glucose as an energy source, and then it will switch to burning fat, predominantly triglycerides, as an energy source. This is the stage we want to reach by using intermittent fasting.

When we burn fat, our body becomes leaner, and we are able to lose weight. Triglyceride levels in the blood are also linked to cardiovascular disease, so the more we are able to reduce these levels naturally, the lower our risk of developing heart-related diseases later in life. This is key for women over 50 as cardiovascular disease is the leading cause of death in women in this age bracket. Intermittent fasting also allows the gastrointestinal (GI) tract to rest and repair itself, which reduces the possibility of cancers and other disorders of the GI tract.

The time period that it takes for the body to reach a stage where it starts to burn fat as fuel is different for everyone, but most research puts it at 10 hours. If there were to be no more fat deposits in your body—which would usually only happen after about 72 hours of zero caloric consumption—your body would start to break down protein for fuel. This process starts with your muscles and then moves to your organs. This is clearly not a stage anyone wants to get to as you are permanently damaging your body by doing so. This process of muscle wastage is the reason that people with severe eating disorders or people who are starving due to a lack of access to food appear gaunt and their muscles appear stringy. The benefit of intermittent fasting is that you are able to access the benefits of fat burning while avoiding the point of muscle wastage. In women over 50, this is especially important as our bone and muscular systems need to remain as strong as possible.

When your body starts to burn fat as fuel, it releases fatty acids called ketones into the bloodstream. Ketones are beneficial to brain health, and their pronounced presence in the body has a number of benefits in preventing disease and improving neural structures, which we will discuss in deeper detail in a later chapter.

The lowering of levels of insulin in our blood when we fast results in an increase in the levels of human growth hormone and norepinephrine in our body. Increasing levels in human growth hormone (HGH) is important for women over 50 as the level of this hormone naturally decreases in our body as we age. Lower levels of HGH result in an increase of fatty tissue and a reduction in muscle mass. Research into HGH also shows that it plays a role in helping people to lose weight without sacrificing muscle. Norepinephrine is a neurotransmitter and stress hormone, which, when released into the body, aids in improving metabolism.

Essentially, our body is always in one of two states, either a fed state where it is producing glucose or fat from food or a fasted state where we are burning stored glucose and fat. If we continuously eat and, therefore, remain in the fed state without ever burning off our glucose and fats stores, we gain weight. This is what makes intermittent fasting such a natural lifestyle. Our bodies are designed to occasionally be in a fasted state. By contrast, our body is not designed to constantly be in a fed state, so if we are snacking every two hours, our body will never burn off our energy stores and it will always just use the incoming food as energy.

Another process that occurs as a result of fasting is autophagy. Autophagy is a natural process whereby the body breaks down damaged or diseased cells and uses that cellular material to produce new, healthy cells. Fasting has been shown to increase the rate of autophagy, therefore increasing the benefits that autophagy provides. Fasting places cells under mild stress, which is actually good for them as it increases their resilience and they are less likely to be damaged or become diseased.

The bulk of laboratory research to date regarding intermittent fasting has been done on animals, but human participants are becoming more common. Real-world results from intermittent fasting speak volumes, though. It is generally difficult to get any human trials approved by the FDA, which is why significant animal subject trials need to be done before moving on to human trials. The difference where this is concerned with intermittent fasting is that human trials, albeit informal and undocumented, have been done for centuries with phenomenal results.

How Fasting Aids in Minimizing Menopausal Symptoms

As an introduction to the concept of menopause—it's astonishing how many women don't really know what is happening in their body—let's briefly discuss the hormonal changes that happen in our bodies and how that impacts weight gain.

When we are in our 40s or 50s, the levels of sex hormones in our body start to decrease. Our ovaries no longer produce hormones like progesterone and estrogen, and we stop releasing eggs from ovaries. As a result of this, menstruation also ceases. This is a process, though, and just because you have missed one menstrual cycle does not necessarily mean you are entering or exiting menopause. In general, health practitioners estimate that if you have not menstruated for 12 months, you can consider yourself as having entered menopause. From a health perspective, it is important to note that menopause is not the only reason that a woman over 50 may miss a period. If the missed menstruation is accompanied by pain or other discomfort or discharge, it is best to consult a doctor to ensure that all is well.

Menopause comes along with some side effects, the severity of which differs from person to person. Some women may only experience one side effect of menopause, while other women may experience all. It is a very unique and individual experience. These side effects include hot flushes, mood changes, night sweats, a decrease in libido, increased risk of heart disease, metabolic changes, and depression and/or anxiety. All of these symptoms are caused by the shift in hormones in your body. The most noted of these symptoms is the change in our metabolism. This can result in menopause-related constipation and, more seriously, weight gain even when we are eating no more than we usually would. It is this symptom that we will focus on here as it so closely relates to our topic. During menopause, we also become more resistant to insulin and our bodies struggle to process refined sugars and carbohydrates. This insulin resistance also results in fatigue and difficulties in sleeping.

Intermittent fasting is, therefore, the perfect solution to balance out our insulin resistance as it is known to make us more sensitive to insulin. This helps our body to break down food properly and not store food as fat unnecessarily.

From a mental health perspective, menopause has a major impact. We are more likely to experience depression, anxiety, brain fog, and mental fatigue. Clinical studies done with animals showed that the impact that fasting has on clearing damaged and diseased brain cells helps to clear brain fog and improve thinking (Bhatia, 2019).

Something that is not often discussed is that from five to 15 years before menopause actually starts, we can be in a phase called perimenopause. This is when your estrogen and progesterone levels start to decrease but are not so low that they are impacting your menstrual cycle. While the two aforementioned hormones are important, there are another three hormones that are starting to fluctuate at that time which also cause problems. These hormones are cortisol, insulin, and oxytocin. In the reverse process of what we have already covered, levels of estrogen and progesterone impact insulin, but insulin also impacts estrogen and progesterone levels. This means that you can just as easily develop insulin in perimenopause as when you are mid-menopause.

As we get older, we also see levels of the stress hormone, cortisol, staying high due to constant stress. When cortisol levels are elevated, so are blood sugar levels, and this results in weight gain specifically around the belly area.

The third hormone being impacted during perimenopause is oxytocin, which is known as the love hormone. It is released when we emotionally bond with others and helps us to feel calmer and less afraid. Oxytocin is the counterweight to cortisol. If we have an increase in oxytocin, then our cortisol levels immediately drop (Cabeca, n.d.).

Menopause can be a scary time in a woman's life. It could be compared to puberty in the context of our body changing, things happening that we don't understand, and often generally feeling overwhelmed. By understanding the chemical processes that are causing your symptoms, they suddenly don't feel quite as insurmountable as they once were. Hormone Replacement Therapy (HRT) is an option for women who are unable to readjust to their new hormone levels. As with anything health-related, though, we would always want to try as many non-invasive means as possible to readjust before turning to medication. Intermittent fasting is definitely an option that should be tried before resorting to HRT.

Weight Loss in Menopausal and Post-Menopausal Women

In 2012, the findings of a study were released, which compared weight loss in groups of menopausal and post-menopausal women. The objective of the study was to compare how body composition and metabolic profile differed in two groups of participants when each group was given a different eating plan to follow. One group was asked to follow an intermittent fasting plan, and the other was asked to follow a continuous eating plan with caloric restrictions (so-called 'normal eating'). The study allowed for the weight that could be regained after ceasing the eating plan by including a stabilization period for each group after their weight-loss period and before the final results were measured. The study, therefore, measured the immediate efficacy of the plan as well as the impact on the body after the plan ceased.

The group on the intermittent fasting plan showed significant decreases in weight, circumference measurements, and body fat measurements. Decreases were also seen in the levels of triglycerides and total cholesterol as well as stabilization of glucose levels (Arguin, 2012). In general, results on intermittent fasting were quicker and longer-lasting than on a continuous eating diet even with caloric intake reductions.

As our bodies tend to react differently to weight loss regimes during menopause, it is important to be patient and stick to your plans. If you have tried fasting in the past and had excellent and fast results but that was before your entered menopause, don't expect the exact same result this time around. You will definitely still lose the weight that you want to if you do what you should be doing, but it may not happen at the rate that you may be used to. If you are fasting with a friend, even if she is also experiencing menopause, do not compare your results to her results. Each individual is different, and that is why it is important to have very specific and measurable goals so that you don't get distracted or lose momentum.

How Else Does Intermittent Fasting Benefit Women Over 50?

Women, in general, have a longer lifespan than men, and as we age, no matter how fit or healthy we are, we are at risk for certain health problems:

- **Breast cancer** occurs when cells in the breast essentially malform and become malignant. It is the most common cancer in women, and more than half of the women diagnosed with cancer are 65 years old or older. Intermittent fasting is known to decrease inflammation in the body. Inflammation is a key precursor to the diagnosis of cancer. Autophagy also ensures that malformed cells are more likely to be destroyed before they become malignant.
- **Osteoporosis** occurs as a result of a reduction in bone density. Bone density reduces with age because our

body slows down the cell renewal process and we cannot replace bone cells at the same rate at which they are breaking down. One in three women over 50 will experience bone breakages due to osteoporosis. Weight loss helps to prevent further breakdown of bone cells, and autophagy also helps to slow the rate of degradation.

- In the U.S., even though seniors only make up 13 percent of the population, they also make up 25 percent of **type 2 diabetes** sufferers. Type 2 diabetes is one of the diseases that, in clinical studies, intermittent fasting has been shown to significantly decrease and, in some situations, reverse.
- **Arthritis** is far more common in women over 50 than men of any age. There are various causes for arthritis including a malfunctioned autoimmune response that results in osteoarthritis. Intermittent fasting improves the functioning of our immune system, which helps to avoid these malfunctioned responses. Overweight arthritis sufferers are more likely to experience additional pain, so

using intermittent fasting to lose weight will reduce your pain as well.

- **Depression** is most diagnosed in women between the ages of 41 and 59. This could have a lot to do with the hormonal changes during menopause, which can be significantly stabilized through intermittent fasting.

When Is Intermittent Fasting Not Good for You?

At the outset, it is important to note that if you have had an unhealthy relationship with food in the past as a result of an eating disorder such as anorexia or bulimia, then you should not attempt an intermittent fasting lifestyle. The process of structuring your eating times may easily cause such a disorder to reoccur. Pregnant or breastfeeding women or women who are trying to get pregnant should also not practice intermittent fasting until they are outside of these periods of time. If you are under a significant amount of stress or experiencing disordered sleeping patterns, you may want to avoid commencing your intermittent fasting journey until you have been able to get those challenges under control. If you are currently underweight (a

BMI of less than 18.5), intermittent fasting is not a good idea.

If you live with any of the following conditions, you can still undertake an intermittent fasting lifestyle, but you should do so after consulting a doctor:

- If you have diabetes type 1 or 2
- If you have elevated uric acid levels or suffer from gout
- If you are on any type of prescription/chronic medication
- If you suffer from chronic heart, liver, or kidney disease

Generally, thanks to the flexible nature of intermittent fasting, most protocols can work around daily stress because if you happen to skip a day, you can always pick it up on another day, so instead of increasing your stress levels, you can reduce your anxiety about not always sticking to your plan.

When deciding whether intermittent fasting is for you, be realistic and be kind to yourself. While it is important to focus on your health, if you feel that you are not mentally prepared to try out a new lifestyle, give yourself some time and set a date in the future when you will start.

While intermittent fasting is very helpful in helping to reduce the symptoms and even reverse certain diseases, it is important to listen to your doctor if you are suffering from any chronic or serious disease, and don't push to start the lifestyle if your doctor advises against it. Your health is the ultimate priority.

People who work in high-stress jobs where decisions are literally life and death—for instance, policemen, firemen, paramedics, and ER doctors—should consider starting intermittent fasting when they are on vacation. This will help to reduce any chance of the cognitive adjustment that happens in the first few days of fasting impacting such duties. Alternatively, people working such jobs could fast on their off days and structure their fast in such a way that they are fasting when they are not working. Professional athletes should work with their dietitians to ensure that their fasting schedule is optimized for their specific energy needs as this differs depending on the type of sport being played. Hydration is also key for athletes, so that should be a major consideration.

This chapter has given you a significant amount of information regarding the science behind intermittent fasting. It is a lot to take in, and it may be wise to reread this chapter at the end of the book again so that you are sure you have absorbed everything. The most important part of any new lifestyle is understanding how it really works, so spend as much time on the concepts we have discussed here as possible. Do additional research if you want to, but make sure that when you start your intermittent fasting lifestyle, you know what is happening inside your body.

Chapter 3: Benefits of Intermittent Fasting for Women Over 50

The benefits of intermittent fasting apply to people of all ages, but there are very specific additional benefits for women over 50. Improvements will be seen in areas of lifestyle, physical health, emotional health, and cognitive ability. As we are all individuals, each person will have a different experience with the benefits we see from fasting. Your focus will likely be on a specific area, and that will be the reason you chose to take on the intermittent lifestyle in the first place. It would stand to reason that your focus would be on the benefits available in that area, but it is important to keep an open mind as weight loss, for instance, is important but overall vitality and wellness are just as important.

Lifestyle Benefits

When compared to other diets, the simplicity of intermittent fasting makes it perhaps the easiest eating protocol through which to experience significant health benefits. Often, the complexity of some eating plans causes people to fail at the first hurdle because as much as they think they understand what they should be doing, they really don't. This results in people going to punishing extremes in order to fulfill what they think they are supposed to be doing and ending up with very disappointing results. Intermittent fasting couldn't be simpler—now you eat and now you don't. Often, special diets can be extremely expensive to follow. You have to purchase special ingredients and eat food that you ordinarily wouldn't. Intermittent fasting is different in that regard too. It costs you absolutely nothing to practice intermittent fasting, and other than a caloric reduction in the case of weight loss and eating as healthy as possible, there is no dictation as to what to eat.

Intermittent fasting is flexible, so it allows you gaps in between to eat the things you enjoy. What is life without an occasional dessert, some chocolate, or pizza? With intermittent fasting, you can have those treats and not feel guilty because when you fast, your body will be burning that treat off. Of course, that is not to say that in every eating window you can binge on every fast food known to mankind. You will still need to eat a healthy diet; you just won't be weighing food and calculating its calorie content all the time.

If you have found an eating plan that you enjoy such as Keto, Paleo, or the like, you can incorporate that with intermittent fasting. There are no other plans available where you can combine two and get even better results. Intermittent fasting is a fantastic addition to other eating plans and does not detract from any other diets (Fung, 2020).

For women over 50, the adjustment to menopause can mean a temporary change in lifestyle. In severe situations, menopause can result in difficulties in relationships with partners and loved ones. Intermittent fasting can help make a big difference in these challenges, and this can be life-changing.

Health Benefits

Cardiovascular health should be a strong focus for people of all ages but even more so for women over 50. The most significant cause of death for women over 50 today is cardiovascular disease. This umbrella term describes all diseases of the heart or the arteries leading to and from the heart. This could include blockages, damage, and deformities in structure. There are several risk factors that contribute to the occurrence of cardiovascular disease including smoking, physical inactivity, genetics, and diet. The latter, however, has been found to be the largest controllable contributor to heart disease.

The most impactful factor where diet is concerned is the types of protein sources that are eaten as well as the types of fats that are consumed. Plant proteins such as beans and legumes have been proven to be a healthier source of protein than animal proteins in general.

Where animal protein is concerned, the leaner the source, the better, and poultry and fish are always healthier options than red meat. The fat component of red meat is another problem where heart disease is concerned, as are other sources of fat such as cooking oils and spreads used for bread. Saturated fats are the types of fats we want to avoid in our diet, and these include animal fat, lard, and tropical oils such as palm oil. Unsaturated fats in small quantities are healthier. Examples of unsaturated fats include avocados, nuts, olive oil, and vegetable oils. When we eat foods in excess of what our body is able to burn, the leftover food forms triglycerides that, at high levels, contribute to the occurrence of cardiovascular disease. When we fast, our body burns triglycerides for energy thereby reducing the levels in our blood and, in turn, reducing our risk of cardiovascular disease.

In the last chapter, we discussed the impact of intermittent fasting on insulin levels. In our eating window, we experience an increase in insulin levels, and when we fast, those levels are decreased. This decrease in insulin results in less food being stored as fat. In animal trials, intermittent fasting has been shown to prevent and reverse Type 2 Diabetes. Another thing that happens when insulin levels decrease is that the FOXO transcription factors, which are known to positively impact metabolism, become more active in the body. This process is also linked to improved longevity and healthy aging.

Another noncommunicable disease that seems to be impacted by intermittent fasting is cancer. Growth Factor 1 (GF1) is a hormone very similar in nature to insulin, and the presence of this hormone is known to be a marker for cancer development. Levels of GF1 are reduced during intermittent fasting.

Women over 50 are twice as likely to develop breast cancer, for instance, and risk factors for other common cancers are also thought to increase when women start to experience the hormonal changes of menopause.

<u>Intermittent fasting is, therefore, an excellent preventative measure for the occurrence of cancer in women over 50.</u>

The increased cell resilience seen in people who regularly fast has been linked to a stronger immune system as well as general faster recovery from illness. The process of building cell resilience through fasting is similar to exercising muscles. The more you undertake regular exercise with periods of rest in between, the stronger your muscles become.

The autophagy process that is triggered by intermittent fasting has been shown to help reduce inflammation in the body as well as oxidative stress, which is primarily responsible for cell damage in the body. Inflammation in various parts of the body has been shown to be present as a precursor to the diagnosis of many different noncommunicable diseases. The diagnosis of noncommunicable diseases is far more common in women over 50 than any other age group. It is, therefore, vital for women in this age group to make use of intermittent fasting and autophagy as an additional preventative measure against the development of noncommunicable diseases.

The Circadian Cycle is the name given to the rhythm created in our body by light and dark (day and night). This natural rhythm controls our need to sleep and eat and has a major impact on our metabolism, cognitive function, and emotional health. It is our internal clock, and when disrupted, it can have devastating effects on our bodies. Intermittent fasting has been shown to help regulate the Circadian Cycle and, if it is out of loop, reset it back to its natural function.

From an evolutionary perspective, our bodies are designed to eat during the day and not to eat at night. This, of course, is the reverse in certain nocturnal mammals who have evolved to reverse that Circadian Cycle due to the availability of prey at night. As modern humans, we have disrupted our Circadian Cycle by not going to sleep when the sun goes down and also continuing to eat well into the night. This impacts our metabolism and our sleeping patterns, resulting in weight gain and sleep disorders such as insomnia. By using intermittent fasting to reset our internal clock to its evolutionary default, we can encourage weight loss by optimizing our metabolism and have a more restful sleep.

In women over 50, this is particularly beneficial. As we age, sleep disorders become more common. We feel tired earlier, experience disturbed sleep, and generally find that we are unable to sleep for as many hours as we once could. This disruption in sleep, of course, has a major impact on our health both physically and mentally. The reason for this change in sleep is due to the reduced levels of Human Growth Hormone (HGH) in our bodies as we age. As we now know, intermittent fasting helps to increase the levels of HGH in our body, thus allowing us to regain a more regular sleeping pattern.

It is important to point out that your last meal of the day should be eaten at least two hours before you go to sleep, and it should be a satisfying but not overly large meal. If you eat too long before you go to bed, you may experience hunger pangs while you sleep that disrupt your sleep. If you eat too large a meal before going to sleep, your body will still be diverting additional blood flow to your stomach to digest its contents, and that will also disrupt your sleep. The importance of a good sleeping pattern cannot be understated as poor sleeping patterns have even been shown to increase the likelihood of the occurrence of certain cancers.

Intermittent fasting has also been shown to improve the regulation of genes that promote liver health and also in the balance of gut bacteria. Gut bacteria play a role in our immune system, and it is vital to keep these gut guests in good shape to optimize your body's defense systems (Kresser, 2019).

Cognitive Functioning Benefits

As you move into your 50s, there are several different effects on your brain health and, as a result, your cognitive functioning. Brain shrinkage automatically occurs as we age, and although it is not something we can avoid, it is certainly something that we can delay and slow down. From a fasting perspective, the process of autophagy, which speeds up during fasting, can help to consume damaged brain cells and use that cellular material to produce new brain cells. This process can help to alleviate the natural brain shrinkage process.

The release of ketones during the burning of fat which occurs during fasting is also highly beneficial to brain health. The enhanced level of ketones helps to protect the brain from the development of epileptic seizures, Alzheimer's Disease, and other neurodegenerative diseases. Of course, as we age, we are also more likely to develop neurodegenerative diseases. Diseases like Alzheimer's and other forms of dementia do have a wide range of risk factors including genetics and smoking. Fasting to enhance autophagy and ketone production is one way that we put up a line of defense against these diseases.

A study conducted on participants over 50, all of whom were already exhibiting some form of impaired cognitive function, showed that by increasing the levels of ketones in the participants' bodies, their cognitive functioning increased within six weeks. It is believed that the reason ketones are so beneficial in increasing cognitive function is due to the fact that they trigger the release of brain-derived neurotrophic factor (BDNF). BDNF helps to strengthen the neural connections in our brain, which are the pathways that our brain uses to transmit thoughts and instructions. BDNF particularly helps to strengthen the pathways that focus on memory and learning. Studies have also shown that intermittent fasting also helps to promote the growth of new nerve cells in the brain.

Intermittent fasting can also help to improve neuroplasticity, which is the brain's natural capability to build new neural pathways. This is imperative in learning as well as in the breaking of habits. When we break bad habits, we actually work to remove the brain's reliance on a commonly used neural pathway and promote the use of a new pathway. Studies in people with brain injuries have shown that intermittent fasting speeds up healing.

Emotional Health

The positive impact of intermittent fasting on our Circadian Cycle also has a knock-on effect on our emotional health. Older adults who are also experiencing sleep disorders are far more likely to develop depression, anxiety, and other emotional disorders. General mood is also impacted by sleep, and lack of proper sleep can cause irritability and general unhappiness in otherwise even-tempered people.

When we practice an intermittent fasting lifestyle, we are taking a significant amount of pressure off ourselves in that we no longer need to concern ourselves with constant meal preparation and structuring our day around food consumption. Until you start practicing an intermittent fasting lifestyle, you will likely not realize how much of your time and mental capacity is dedicated to thinking about food. When that pressure is taken off you because you know exactly when you will be eating and when you will not be eating, a weight is lifted off your shoulders.

Intermittent fasting is an all-around mood enhancer with the added benefit of a feeling of achievement when you are able to stick to your new lifestyle because it is so much easier to achieve than most eating plans or diets.

When we enter menopause, our risk of developing depression and anxiety increases, as do the mood swings we experience that may be completely alien to us. Suddenly feeling completely out of control of moods and emotions when, for most of our lives we have been stable, can be very frightening. Intermittent fasting stabilizes the levels of hormones to bring our emotions back within our control.

The emotional impact of menopause can be quite significant, and although intermittent fasting will definitely help, it is important to keep in mind that sometimes we need professional help to deal with any depression or anxiety that we are dealing with as a result of menopause. If you have suffered from any emotional disorders in the past, in fact, it is a good idea to discuss your options with your doctor as soon as you become aware that you are entering menopause. Even if you are already taking medication such as antidepressants, the changes in your hormone levels may cause them to become less effective. Our emotional health is vital to our physical health, and it is very important for us to focus on this at this time in our lives. In the past, you may have pushed your emotions down in order to be able to be of service to others. As women, this is not uncommon. We cannot help others if we are struggling ourselves, though, so this is the time to make yourself a priority and make sure that you get the help you need so that you can live your best life.

In this chapter, we have covered the lifestyle, physical health, cognitive functioning, and emotional health benefits of intermittent fasting. You may be surprised at just how impactful fasting is on our body and on our lives overall. Understanding these benefits is a good way to motivate yourself along the way. When you have started your journey and you are seeing these benefits in your life, come back to this chapter and see how many of the listed benefits you can check off as having materialized in your life thanks to your commitment to an intermittent fasting lifestyle.

Chapter 4: Intermittent Fasting Protocols

One of the best aspects of the intermittent fasting lifestyle is that it is extremely flexible. The basic dynamic is that you have an eating window and a fasting window, but the way that you structure those windows is really completely up to you. Depending on your own lifestyle, your family structure, and work obligations, you can structure your fasting according to several different protocols or adjust one of these protocols to suit you. You may want to try more than one protocol for a little while and then pick the one that suits you best. It is going to be a very individual decision and based on what feels right for you and which protocol gives you the best results.

The protocols we will discuss here are dual in nature. All can be practiced as pure intermittent fasting protocols—fast without eating and then eat without changing what you eat, except for reducing calories for weight loss and maintaining a healthy diet. Some protocols have been adopted by specific fitness experts, and they have added their own twists to the protocols. It is our intention to provide you with as much knowledge as possible so that you can make your own decisions about which protocol works for you.

The 16:8 Protocol

We briefly discussed this protocol earlier in the book. The general idea is that the first number in the ratio is your fasting window represented in hours and the second number is your eating window, also represented in hours. This protocol is the most popular as it is the easiest to achieve considering we are already sleeping for eight hours. This method is particularly good to help obese people lose weight and reduce their blood pressure quickly. This protocol is also very good for beginner intermittent fasters as it is easy to adapt to. This method is also known as the Leangains Protocol and was made popular by fitness expert Martin Berkhan.

You can fit two or three meals into your eating window, but the recommendation is a light lunch to break the fast and then a more substantial dinner. Women tend to do better on shorter fasts, so this protocol is ideal for women over the age of 50. Many experts recommend that women actually limit their fast to 14 or 15 hours (Gunnars, 2020). Again, this is completely an individual choice, and as long as you are able to cope well and you are not seeing any negative side effects, the length of your fast is completely up to you.

The 20:4 Protocol

This protocol is also called the Warrior Diet and was developed by fitness expert Ori Hofmekler. The protocol involves a 20-hour fasting window and a four-hour eating window. The eating window should preferably be at night to work with this protocol, and the meal is supposed to represent a 'feast' at the end of the 'battle.' Although the fasting period is so long on this protocol, some versions do allow for a small amount of snacking during the fasting window. Raw fruit and vegetables are allowed as snacks, so essentially, it is not true fast. Very little research has been done into this fasting protocol, and it is not recommended as an appropriate protocol for those who are just starting their intermittent fasting journey. The Warrior Diet also diverges from traditional intermittent fasting by dictating the types of foods which should be eaten. These include foods that are similar to how they occur in nature, which is much like the protocols on the Paleo diet.

The other option with a 20:4 fast is to not look at it from the Warrior diet perspective but rather from a pure intermittent fasting perspective. In other words, following the time allocations without eating during the fasting window and eating normally during the eating window. Keeping your eating window at night does make sense with this protocol as you could have a good meal when you break your fast and then time it so that you are going to sleep quite soon after you finish eating. This could then count as your next fast period.

Whole Day Fast

As the name of this protocol suggests, the fast window is 24 hours long. The Whole Day Fast protocol is more of an umbrella term for various fasting methods than a protocol in and of itself. The protocol can be implemented by fasting as little as two days per month or as much as twice per week. This method has been popularized in the Eat-Stop-Eat diet, in which two days per week are 24-hour fasts.

The 5:2 method, which is also called The Fast Diet and was made popular by British journalist Michael Mosley, dictates fasting for two days out of the week, and on those two fast days, caloric consumption should be no more than 600 calories. The 5:2 method is one of the few intermittent fasting protocols that calls for severe caloric control and is clearly aimed specifically at those wanting to lose weight. The other five days of the week do not call for any major caloric reduction other than healthy eating choices.

The alternate-day fasting method also falls under the 'whole day fast' umbrella and promotes fasting every other day of the week (Kresser, 2019). There are several versions of the alternate-day fast as well, and some of those dictate a caloric consumption of no more than 500 calories on fast days.

The 6:1 Fast

This protocol means that for one 24-hour period in a week, you eat nothing at all. So, you could start with breakfast and then fast for 24 hours until the next breakfast. You definitely want to keep yourself well hydrated during this time as you will be having no food at all. Other beverages with no calorie content are also permitted.

The Keto Derivative Fast

This protocol combines the Keto diet (designed to bring you into a ketosis state faster) and intermittent fasting. In this protocol, the hours are fixed as the eating window is from 11 am to 6 pm. It also does fasting a little differently as it dictates what you should eat—no heavy carbohydrates like bread or pasta—and even in which order you should eat food groups. It suggests that vegetables should be eaten first and protein second. Cutting out carbohydrates completely can induce brain fog, so attempt this protocol with caution, especially if you are fasting for the first time.

Spontaneous Fasting

In this protocol, you essentially fast when you feel like it and when it is convenient for you. While the structure that is so beneficial to traditional intermittent fasting regimes is missing from this protocol, it has still shown benefits. Essentially, the idea is that you will use intermittent fasting when it is convenient for you. Perhaps you are going on a trip and won't have easy access to food or you are going to be too busy at work to grab lunch (Gunnars, 2020). There is a debate about whether this can really be called a protocol as such since you are not allocating a fasting window or an eating window. It is more like skipping meals when convenient.

Of course, it is entirely possible to use this method in the same manner that you would other protocols but without planning. For instance, you may find that by 10 am on a weekday, a new deadline has suddenly cropped up and you make the decision that you won't have time to eat so you are going to fast until dinner at 8 pm. You will certainly get the benefits of the fast period if you stick to not eating anything and only taking in zero-calorie beverages. This protocol is not going to work if you are trying to lose weight though, as you will need to be consistent with your fasting. If you don't make a commitment to include fasting in your lifestyle every week in some way, one could also wonder how likely you would be to fast at all.

Crescendo Method

In this method, fasting is conducted on alternate days (i.e. Monday, Wednesday, and

Friday), and the fast window on each of these days is 12 - 16 hours. It is recommended to start on a 12-hour fast and work your way up to 16 hours.

This is quite handy if you work outside of the home and spend your weekends being social and visiting with friends and family as it gives you the opportunity to fast during the workweek and still enjoy your weekends without fasting. You could, of course, just fast for a slightly shorter period on the weekend day as well and fast for longer during the week.

Selecting a Protocol

Choosing which intermittent fasting method to go with really depends on your goals. If you are predominantly looking to lose weight, the 16:8 method has been shown to provide good weight loss results; however, this may be because it is easier to stick to than some of the other protocols. The latter is a very important point to consider. If you are wanting to lose weight, you need to comply with three factors:

- Your calorie intake must be lower than your calorie output. In other words, you must practice a caloric deficit.

- You must include exercise in your lifestyle. This is the best way to ensure a caloric deficit without seriously reducing the amount of food you eat— eat less but also burn more.
- You must be consistent. This is key to any weight loss regime as there is no eating plan on earth that will allow you to lose the weight you want to in a few days and keep it off.

While some intermittent fasting protocols will likely help you shed weight faster, you will only keep that weight off if you are consistent in following the plan. <u>Drastic weight loss over a short period of time is not healthy for anyone and certainly not for women over 50.</u> Everyone is different, and our weight loss challenges also lay in different areas. For some, the issue may lay in overeating at night, just before you go to sleep. Due to the natural slowing of our metabolism when we sleep and the fact that we are not burning any calories, eating a large meal late at night or midnight snacking could be a major cause of weight gain.

You can always change the protocol you choose as nothing is set in stone. Select a plan you believe that you can stick to and one that matches your lifestyle. Ideally, start shorter and work your way up. Not only does this give you a sense of achievement by encouraging success on shorter fasts first, but it also helps you to ease your body into the idea of fasting. This makes it easier to work through the common side effects that initially crop up when you start fasting like headaches and constipation, which we will discuss in the next chapter.

Extended Fasting

Extended fasting is a major talking point in the intermittent fasting community. Essentially, a fast can be considered as extended if it goes on for longer than 48 consecutive hours. Opinions and research on how healthy this is differ, and it may just come down to the individual and what they are able to cope with. Of course, our aversion to extended fasts as a society may just be formed around the general fallacy that we hold onto that we need regular, significant amounts of food to survive. In truth, as long as we stay hydrated, there is really no problem with going without eating for 48 hours. When we are ill with gastro or similar stomach issues and we feel nauseous and have no appetite, we easily go without eating, so to choose to do so when we are well is not really all that different.

In general, extended fasting is not recommended for women over 50 if the individual is new to fasting. If the individual has been fasting for a long period already, continuing to do so will likely not have a major negative impact.

<u>If you are a first-time faster and also a woman over the age of 50, it is important to build your fasting periods up by starting at 10 - 16 hours and moving up from there if you wish to try an extended fast.</u> Always check with your healthcare provider before attempting an extended fast and ensure that you take a good multivitamin and stay hydrated.

One of the biggest risks in extended fasts is refeeding syndrome. This occurs when food is reintroduced to a body that has been without it for an extended period of time. Refeeding syndrome usually only occurs in people who have not eaten for 14 days or more but this is completely an individual experience and depending on your own metabolism and body structure, you could experience the syndrome after a far shorter period of fasting. Refeeding syndrome causes a shift in the body's fluids and minerals and can, if left untreated, lead to death. It is for this reason that people who have had no access to food, including eating disorder patients, are treated by slowly reintroducing nutritional fluids and eventually solid food.

If you are attempting an extended fast, it is interesting to note that hunger tends to recede after the second day of not eating. As a general rule, if you fast more often, you will see a reduction in appetite. This is due to a break that occurs in the insulin resistance cycle and a reduction in the levels of insulin. Your body's response to this is to decrease your appetite but maintain general energy expenditure levels (Fung, 2016). This reduction in appetite is a chemical process and has nothing to do with the size of your stomach. You have likely heard people talk about the shrinking and stretching of the stomach; however, there is no medical backing to support the idea that your stomach ever undergoes a change in size after adulthood. The only way to make your stomach smaller is through surgery, and this is done only when a morbidly obese person is otherwise unable to control their eating. What actually happens is that when your relationship with food changes, you experience psychological changes and chemical changes within your body that are the true root of eating more or less. It has nothing to do with the size of the stomach organ. Reduction in appetite happens when your levels of the hunger hormone change and can also be attributed to a difference in emotional or psychological reactions to food and eating.

One of the longest recorded fasts in history lasted 362 days! While we certainly don't recommend that and, honestly, wonder how that is even humanly possible, it certainly is a testament to the human ability to go without food for long periods of time. A study that was performed around extended fasting admitted subjects to a hospital for 14-day fasts. The subjects were all predominantly obese and needed to urgently lose weight for health reasons. Besides seeing significant health improvements and weight loss after the 14-day period, researchers actually had several participants request that they be booked back into the study to continue fasting.

In this chapter, we have discussed all of the intermittent fasting protocols that have emerged in the last few years. Some of these are simply derivatives of other protocols and include very specific eating plans that are not essential to intermittent fasting. It is recommended that you try one or two different protocols before deciding on a particular method. One method might work relatively well for you but another method may knock it out of the park in terms of the benefits you experience. As long as you are fasting, it doesn't really matter how you fast, so you have free rein to try as many different protocols as you wish before nailing yourself down to one.

Chapter 5: Practical Tips for Intermittent Fasting and Overcoming Challenges

While intermittent fasting is one of the easier dietary lifestyles to implement, there are ways that you can make your transition easier and overcome some of the challenges related to intermittent fasting. Knowing what challenges you can expect already puts you in a more empowered space as you won't be surprised when you experience a challenge in the first few days of fasting. It often helps to be in touch with someone who is an experienced faster so that they can give you real-world feedback about how they felt when they started fasting and what they did to overcome the challenges.

Social media is quite a powerful tool for this as there are now support groups and forums that you can join in order to speak with others who are committing to the intermittent fasting journey. Support like this really does make a huge difference, especially if you are starting out on your intermittent fasting journey on your own. Having someone to bounce questions off and get feedback from is invaluable. It's also great to have a cheerleader of sorts—someone who you can count on to motivate you when times get tough and celebrate with you when you achieve your goals.

Plan for Success and Commit to Yourself

Once you are in a good rhythm with regard to your intermittent fasting, you will find it easy to work around your fasting and eating windows. At the very beginning of your journey, though, it is important to plan for success. Once you have selected a specific protocol to match your lifestyle, it is important to plan a month or so in advance to see if there are days when your chosen protocol may not work for you and plan around that.

As an example, perhaps you have chosen the 16:8 protocol, and you have decided to practice it from Monday to Friday and give yourself a break on the weekends, but you have a regular Friday breakfast appointment with a friend that has become a tradition. Instead of ignoring the fact that this clashes with your new lifestyle, plan around that in advance to avoid having to make last-minute decisions. You could either decide to skip fasting on a Friday and fast, instead, from Monday to Thursday and then on a Saturday or you could contact your friend and ask if you could move your breakfast dates to a Saturday morning instead.

While this may seem a small issue to be focusing on, it is actually extremely important. If you want to maintain consistency, the enemy of that is going to be issues that crop up that you haven't planned for. Similarly, consider what your family life looks like. Do you usually eat breakfast with your family in the morning? If so, you may need to explain to them that you are going to be embarking on a new lifestyle that will require you to skip breakfast. If they rely on you to make their breakfast, this is a good opportunity to change that. Cereals and toast are easy enough for most people to make on their own. If you feel that you may be tempted by being around your family when they are eating breakfast, turn their breakfast time into your exercise time.

Have a plan for other situations that may crop up. What will you do if a colleague or friend invites you to lunch outside of your eating window? What if a colleague has a birthday, and during your fasting window, you find a delicious piece of chocolate cake planted on your desk?

Having plans for situations like this will help you avoid faltering on your intermittent fasting lifestyle. You will also feel more confident if you feel that you are in control of your lifestyle and that you are able to make good decisions on the spur of the moment because you have planned for them. A lot of these types of situations can be helped by sharing your plans with your family, close friends, and coworkers.

If you are specifically using intermittent fasting to lose weight, be sure to throw out your scale and whip out your measuring tape instead. In fact, in all weight loss endeavors, regardless of the method you are trying, you should never rely on a scale to determine your progress. The scale lies, perhaps unintentionally, but it does not tell you anything about what you really want to know. You want to know how much fat you have lost. When you weigh yourself, you are including water and muscle. If you are increasing your water consumption for fasting, you are weighing all of that water, and if you are including muscle-toning, then you are also weighing additional muscle that you may have built during exercise. The only way to get a true reflection of your progress is by taking your measurements.

A journal, whether a book or digitally-based, and a calendar are two very helpful tools in intermittent fasting. Use your journal to write down your goals and your reasons for starting intermittent fasting. When drafting your goals, be sure to use the SMART criteria to ensure that your goals are setting you up for success and not failure. SMART goals are:

- **Specific:** State exactly what you want to achieve. Saying, "I want to lose weight" is not sufficient. Rather say, "I want to lose 10 pounds," or even better, to avoid the scale, "I want to lose ___ inches."
- **Measurable:** How are you going to determine how far along you have come in your journey to reaching your goals? You need to be able to measure your progress not only so that you can restructure if you need to but also so that you can celebrate your wins.
- **Achievable:** Don't set goals that are impossible to achieve because you are only setting yourself up for failure and

disappointment. Be kind to yourself; you are already embarking on a journey that many don't have the courage to embrace.

- **Realistic:** Ensure that you are being realistic with yourself about what your capabilities, current ailments, and other lifestyle restrictions might mean to your goals. While you don't want to be too hard on yourself, you do need to push a bit to achieve what you want.

- **Time-bound:** This criterion goes hand-in-hand with measurability. You must set a specific time period for when you want to have reached your goals so that you can accurately measure your progress.

Setting goals for your intermittent fasting journey is important and will be based around your reasons for starting the journey. If weight loss is your main goal, then you will very likely structure your goals around how many pounds or inches you want to lose in a certain period of time. If your main reason for starting fasting is to reduce the effects of an illness, you could structure your goals around which symptoms of your illness you would like to see reduced or perhaps by a reduction in the medication you need to take for that illness. Setting SMART goals is a balance because you want to push yourself enough to make it a challenge and not so easy to achieve that there is no point in setting the goal at all. But you also need to be realistic about time, your personal circumstances, and your current state of health.

Share Your Plans

Your intermittent fasting lifestyle is a very personal choice, but it will have some impact on the lives of those around you. When you make the decision to embark on this journey, it is important to explain to those who are close to you exactly what you will be doing and why. Be prepared for some surprise or adverse reactions. Don't let this put you off; you have done your homework, and you can explain the science behind intermittent fasting to these people if necessary. Ultimately, this is your choice, and you only really need to share your plans so that others are able to support you if they so wish and not for their approval.

Your family will be the most impacted by your decision, but they will also likely receive the most benefit from your new lifestyle.

Intermittent fasting will improve your mood and give you more energy. Its multiple health benefits should also be important to your family as they should want you to be as healthy as possible. Ideally, it would be beneficial to have your partner practice intermittent fasting with you as this will make things far easier at home. If they are not ready to try or are not interested in intermittent fasting, though, don't let this put you off. It is absolutely possible to still be successful in this new lifestyle without others in your home also embarking on it.

Your close friends will be the second group to be impacted by your new lifestyle but only if your interactions often involve food. Your coworkers will be the least impacted by your decision, but if there is a culture of eating at work, it will be important to share your plans there as well.

By involving those who love and care for you, you are more likely to stick to your intermittent fasting lifestyle as you will have others holding you accountable. At the end of the day, though, you are doing this for your own benefit, and there is really no need for approval or agreement from others. Thankfully, if you are a woman over 50, you

<u>have likely already reached a point in your life where you don't seek outside approval anymore and the opinions of others matter very little in the grand scheme of things.</u>

If you find it difficult to get support from those in your life, use online options like internet support groups to find people who will support you. It is quite likely that you are able to achieve your goals on your own without external support, but it is also helpful to have someone to chat with when you are uncertain about an aspect of fasting or to celebrate with when you start achieving your goals.

Plan Your Meals

By choosing intermittent fasting as a lifestyle, you have already taken a lot of pressure off yourself by structuring your eating window and eliminating at least one meal. You can take this further and increase your chances of being successful by planning your meals and prepping your food beforehand. This is especially important if you are aiming for weight loss as you will need to keep your calories down to a certain level. You don't have to plan your meals too far in advance—a week at a time is more than sufficient. If you have, for instance, decided to fast between Monday and Friday, set aside some time on a Sunday afternoon for meal preparation for the week.

This is especially important for the first meal of your eating window. You are likely going to be hungry and you don't want to eat an enormous meal to break your fast as that will only leave you feeling overly full and possibly a little ill. Plan a few light meals for your first meal of the day such as nutritious sandwiches, wraps, or salads with protein. You want to feel satisfied so that you can make it through to your next meal without gorging yourself.

In the last chapter, we will provide you with specific food suggestions, but in general, the key is to significantly increase your fruit and vegetable intake and include healthy protein and fat choices.

Exercising While Fasting

Exercise is not only important in a generally healthy lifestyle, but it is also vital for weight loss. If you are already involved in some form of exercise, you can continue with your routine while fasting. You do not need to eat before you exercise as you will then burn stored energy reserves including fat, which is ideal. This is a personal choice, though; if you feel light-headed when exercising without having eaten, you can move the time that you exercise to just after your first light meal in your eating window. By doing so, you can also limit your appetite and further speed up your metabolism for the balance of your eating window.

Whether or not you choose to eat before exercising, you must ensure that you stay hydrated. A lot of the water we consume actually comes from our food, so it is much easier to become dehydrated during exercise when fasting. You should also watch your sodium intake and ensure that your levels are high enough as you will lose sodium through perspiration during exercise.

Exercise for women over 50 should be structured based on your current fitness levels. If you have been an athlete or consistent exerciser your entire life, then you will likely need to make very few changes. _If your exercise journey starts with your intermittent fasting journey then, as a woman over 50, you will need to make some adjustments._

Increased physical activity for women over 50 has far-reaching benefits and not just for weight loss. Exercise helps your body to minimize the side effects of menopause including hot flashes, joint pain, and sleeping problems. Belly fat is a major issue in our 50s, and there are certain exercises that are perfect for targeting this area. The perfect exercise regime for a woman over 50 includes the following components:

- Stretching exercises
- Aerobic or cardiovascular exercises
- Strength or muscle-training exercises

The reason for including these three types of exercise is to work the different areas of your body and maximize the health and weight loss benefits.

Stretching exercises include yoga and pilates, which help to strengthen core muscles and increase the flexibility of muscles. For women over 50, the biggest benefit of this type of exercise is the increase in joint strength. It also helps to reduce the possibility of injury during other types of exercise.

Aerobic or cardiovascular exercises work the large muscles in your body and are beneficial to your cardiovascular system. Such exercises include jogging, cycling, walking, and dancing. As a woman over 50, you may already be suffering from some form of joint weakness if you have not exercised throughout your life. In this case, you could start with more stretching exercises and lower impact cardio exercises such as swimming or cycling. Once you have strengthened your joints, you may be able to move on to other types of cardio exercise like jogging.

It is important not to overdo your cardio exercise if you are new to it. The "talk test" is the best way to gauge whether you are exercising at the right level. You should be able to carry on a conversation with ease while you are exercising. If you find it very difficult to do so, you may want to reduce the intensity of your exercise until you are able to speak easily and then step it up slightly.

Strength training helps with toning, improves your strength and posture, and reduces the chance that you will experience a lower back injury. Small hand weights are the easiest way to strength train at home. If you are using gym facilities, they will likely have a wide range of machines for weight training. Start small, though, and don't overdo it as you will only injure yourself. Start with a weight that you can easily handle for eight repetitions then increase the size of the weight until you can do 12 repetitions at a time.

The key to any exercise is starting small and working your way up. You should feel invigorated and full of energy when you are finished exercising, not exhausted, light-headed, or ill. Choose an exercise that you enjoy and you will be more likely to stick to it. Just as with intermittent fasting, you should choose a method that fits your lifestyle and will not take much additional effort in order to accomplish. Choose a method of exercise that can either be done anywhere or that does not take too much of a trip to get to. The more effort required in actually achieving a routine, the more likely you are to find excuses to avoid it.

Formal exercises do not need to be the only form of exercise you get. It is possible to increase your activity levels in your daily life with a few different choices. Walk your dog more often, take the stairs rather than the elevator, or park a little further from the mall or office entrance. Small changes like this can make a huge difference. There are many tools for measuring our exercise achievements including pedometers (which count our steps) built into cell phones and watches (WebMD, n.d.).

Even if weight loss is not your main goal, you definitely still want to include exercise in your fasting regime for the health benefits. If you are not trying to burn calories, your exercise can be slightly less structured. As long as you are increasing your activity levels, you will see the benefits of additional exercise.

Water Is Your Friend

A lot of the fluid we take in comes from our food, so when we restrict our food intake to specific periods, we put ourselves at risk of dehydration. Thankfully, this is easily remedied by increasing our water intake. In general, we should be drinking about eight glasses of water per day, but this can be different from person to person and also depends on how much exercise you do and the weather. When it is warmer, we tend to perspire more and, therefore, lose water at a faster rate, so we need to increase our water intake in summer. Water is beneficial not only because it keeps us hydrated but also because it is a vital part of many body processes as well as the functioning of organs.

Drinking water while you are fasting can also help to fight any hunger pangs you may experience. It's also a great way to distract yourself if you are struggling to stick to your fasting window at the beginning of your intermittent fasting journey.

If you aren't a major fan of plain water, you can infuse it with flavors such as lemon, lime, cucumber, and mint to make it more palatable to you. Buy yourself a water-infuser to use at home, though, as flavored store-bought water often contains other additives and has a calorie content. Another option for beverages during your fasting period is tea or coffee. Ideally, you don't want to add sugar or milk to these beverages, but if you are unable to drink plain tea or coffee, add a tiny amount of sugar and nonfat milk.

Green tea is a phenomenal option as a beverage during fasting. It tastes just fine without any additions, and it is packed with antioxidants. Some resources claim that zero-sugar sodas are acceptable to drink when fasting. This is definitely highly debatable as ideally, we would like to not drink sodas at all. The preservatives and additives in soda make it a poor choice where beverages are concerned.

Less in Means Less Out

You would be forgiven for assuming we are referring to calories here. Actually, though, we are referring to your bowel movements. This is an important consideration when fasting as it is one of the challenges that we don't always expect or plan for. If your eating pattern changes, so will the pattern related to your intestinal function and, hence, your bowel movements. It may take some time for your body to settle into a new routine, and while you wait for this to happen, you may experience a period of constipation. You can get yourself through this by drinking more water and eating high-fiber foods. If this doesn't make enough of a difference and you end up experiencing pain and bloating, a mild laxative should do the trick in getting things back to normal. Magnesium supplements are also very helpful in regulating bowel movements, and they have the added benefit of being very important in the life of women over 50 as this is the time you are likely to experience more bone and muscle issues.

As we get older, our bowel movements naturally change and what is normal for one person may not be normal for another.

Menopause can also cause constipation, so if you are embarking on an intermittent fasting journey and already experiencing some level of menopausal constipation, be prepared to work through this. The good news is that constipation related to fasting will pass very quickly.

Headaches and Other Side Effects

It is very common to experience headaches in the first few days of fasting. This is nothing to be concerned about and is your body's natural reaction to a change in the sodium levels in your body. This happens due to the change in your food intake. A small amount of salt and a good supply of water can often help to reduce or minimize the severity of these headaches as the salt will replace the electrolytes, which can be the cause of headaches.

Heartburn, dizziness, and muscle cramps can also be experienced in the first few days of a new intermittent fasting journey.

Dizziness can be caused by dehydration or a low salt level, which can be remedied by drinking a broth or mineral water. Dizziness could also be as a result of low blood pressure. Fasting helps to reduce blood pressure, so if you are taking medication for hypertension (high blood pressure), then that additional reduction can result in your blood pressure being too low. If you believe this to be the case, consult your doctor to see if you can reduce your dosage. Hypertension is very common in women over 50, so the added benefit of decreasing blood pressure is particularly helpful to this age group.

Heartburn can be experienced during fasting especially if you eat a particularly large meal to break your fast. If you stick to lighter meals and ensure that you stay upright for at least 30 minutes after eating (don't go and have a nap right after lunch), you will reduce your chances of experiencing heartburn. As with all other side effects of fasting, your body will begin to adjust within a few days, and these issues will usually correct themselves without outside intervention.

Muscle cramps are most often caused by a lack of magnesium. You can correct this by taking a supplement or soaking in a bath with Epsom salts.

Stay Busy

Particularly in the first few days of fasting, you may find yourself thinking about food more often, and this leads to you thinking that you are hungrier than you actually are. If, before you started your intermittent fasting journey, you were prone to boredom eating, this point is going to be particularly important for you. Have some activities planned ahead that will distract you from the fact that you are not eating. It is preferable to make these high-interest activities such as learning something new or working on projects that take a lot of focus. If you just watch television or chat with a friend, you are likely to still have a lot of brainpower left for obsessing about food. This is another reason why, if you work outside the home, you may find it more beneficial to fast on days when you are working. If you are focusing on your work, it makes it easier to forget that you are in a fasting window and just move on with your day.

The phrase "mind over matter" is very pertinent to hunger. Waves of hunger actually pass very easily and a simple distraction, drinking water, or meditating for a minute will usually help you get past this easily.

Remember why you embarked on this journey in the first place. Think of all of the benefits that you are receiving from fasting. Visualize yourself receiving those benefits—achieving your weight goals, increased energy levels, increased longevity, a better immune system, and an all-around better mood. Surely, a small hunger pang is not worth risking all of those benefits?

If it helps, think about your family. Consider how, by fasting, you are increasing the likelihood that you will get to spend more time with them. Everyone's motivation will be different so find yours and hold on to it. The hunger will subside. Remind yourself that you can eat, just not at that very moment. Also keep in mind that just because you are not physically taking in food, that doesn't mean your body isn't 'eating.' In fact, while you fast, your body is feasting on your fat deposits (Fung, 2020).

In this chapter, we have provided you with real-world tips on what challenges to expect in your intermittent fasting journey and also how to best overcome these challenges. Compared to other weight loss regimes, intermittent fasting certainly has the least negative side effects, and they are easy to overcome. <u>The key is to know that they are coming and preempt them so that you are not caught off guard and overwhelmed in the moment.</u>

Chapter 6: Fasting-Friendly Foods and Recipes

While intermittent fasting does not dictate which foods you should or shouldn't eat during your eating window, there are certainly foods that are preferable. <u>Due to the fact that you are restricting your eating to a specific time, it is important to eat a healthy, well-balanced diet during your eating window to avoid experiencing a deficiency in any of the major nutrient groups.</u>

The recipes that we have chosen to include in this chapter are specifically selected to include foods that will assist you in your fasting window. We have included the nutritional information on each recipe including the number of calories (if you are on a weight loss regime), carbohydrates, fats, fiber, protein, and salt. Salt is required in our diet to act as an electrolyte, but it is harmful in excess, so it is important to track your salt intake. Keep in mind that there is hidden sodium in almost everything.

We have also included a section in each recipe where we tell you beforehand if you need any special equipment for the recipe. All the recipes are adjustable, though, so be sure to have a look at the suggestions and variation notes at the end of each recipe for ways that you can change it up to suit you.

Beverages

During your fasting window, water, coffee, and tea without additives are best to maintain your hydration levels. Cinnamon and licorice teas have appetite suppressant properties that can help you get through your fasting window.

During your eating window, you can spread that out a little but still keep your eye on sugar levels in store-bought drinks as even fruit juices contain very high levels of sugar and other additives. Coffee in moderation is actually very healthy. It improves concentration and also helps to activate the liver to repair the damage done to that organ.

Suggested Foods for Your Eating Window

Foods that are rich in fiber make you feel full for longer. They also help to counter any constipation you may experience in the early days of fasting. Examples of high-fiber foods include fruits, vegetables, nuts, and beans. Raspberries are especially high in fiber and easy to snack on. Lentils are also very high in fiber and, in addition, are a good source of protein and iron. Cruciferous vegetables such as cauliflower, broccoli, and Brussels sprouts are packed with fiber.

Foods that are rich in protein are great for your eating window as they also leave you feeling fuller for longer and are especially beneficial if you are weight training. Examples of protein-rich foods include tofu, fish, meat, legumes, and nuts. A healthy diet includes as little red meat as possible. The excessive consumption of red meat has been linked to the development of several noncommunicable diseases including heart disease, diabetes, and hypertension.

If you are not able to completely remove animal protein from your diet (or prefer not to), try and keep it down to a minimum. Poultry and fish are far better options than red meat, while plant-based proteins are your healthiest option. A cup of lentils contains about half the amount of protein as a cup of red meat, so in order to take in the same amount of protein, you will need to double your portion. That may sound like a problem, but with plant-based proteins, it isn't as they are packed with so many other vitamins and minerals that the additional serving is worth it.

Another excellent plant-based protein option is seitan. Known as "wheat meat," seitan can be cooked the same way you would a meat dish as it has the same consistency. Soybeans are an excellent source of isoflavones, which are known to inhibit the damage done to cells by the sun and promote anti-aging (definitely a huge benefit for women over 50!).

Salmon is one of the healthiest animal proteins to consume as it contains a high amount of omega fatty acids, which are beneficial to women over 50 in aiding the maintenance of brain health. Always choose wild-caught salmon over the farmed variety, though, as farmed salmon are given antibiotics to prevent disease and have been proven to be far less nutritious than wild-caught salmon.

Unless you are specifically following an eating plan that excludes carbohydrates, there is no need to avoid them when you are practicing intermittent fasting. Whole grain breads and wraps are a quick and easy option for carbohydrates that you will be able to easily digest to provide fuel for exercise. Potatoes are also an easily digestible carbohydrate and a good meal to have with a protein source after exercise. When potato cools, it forms a resistant starch and contains prebiotics that assist with the bacteria in our gut that play a role in our immune system. Other examples of similarly digested carbohydrates with prebiotics include artichokes, apples, bananas, and asparagus. Non-carbohydrate prebiotic sources include garlic, leeks, onions, swiss chard, and spinach.

It is not uncommon for intermittent fasters to experience deficiencies in calcium and vitamin D. The predominant reason for this is that both calcium and vitamin D are most commonly consumed through dairy products, and we usually eat those products during breakfast. If we are timing our fast to not consume breakfast, then many of the dairy products we would usually consume in that meal (along with vitamin D and calcium) is missed as well.

Again, this is not anything that should put us off fasting as all we need to do is be strategic enough about including those items in our meals elsewhere. Besides dairy products, kale, tofu, and soy are also excellent sources of calcium and vitamin D.

Another component of dairy that we may be missing out on is vitamin K. Prunes are particularly high in vitamin K as well as fiber. Vitamin K is essential for bone health, which is an area of concern as we age. The additional fiber is another bonus.

Fats have a bad reputation and one that is not always deserved. Low-fat is not always the best option, particularly if the low-fat option contains saturated fats. We need fat in our diet, but we do need to be careful about which fats we choose. For frying, you don't want to heat your oil until it starts smoking as this creates carcinogenic (cancer-causing) properties. Ghee, clarified butter, is an option that has the highest smoking point.

In order to maintain your gut health while you fast and avoid menopausal constipation as an added benefit, you need to include probiotics, which are an important part of the fasting regime. The best sources of probiotics are kefir, kombucha, and kraut. Yogurt can be a source of probiotics, but it depends on how it is made. Highly processed yogurt will retain a very low number of probiotics, so it is far easier to eat a pure source such as one of the aforementioned. Probiotic supplements are readily available but, as with anything that your body needs, it is far more effective to take it in through food.

Whole grains are always a far better option than refined grains, and the portions of the grain that are removed in the refining process are actually the most nutritious. Whole grains are also more filling than refined grains and contain more fiber. Some examples of whole grains include spelt, amaranth, millet, farro, bulgur, and sorghum (Rizzo, 2018).

Barley and oatmeal contain beta-glucan, which is a type of fiber that helps to control blood sugar. When our blood sugar is stable, we get hungry less quickly.

Herb maca is a superfood that is phenomenally effective in women over 50 in regulating hormones as well as insulin and blood sugar levels. It is a tuber that is very similar in taste to a radish and originates from Peru. Maca is sold in a powder form and can be included in smoothies, mixed in with yogurt, or dissolved in tea. A clinical study was done to determine the real-world benefits of maca on menopausal women. Over a period of four months, a group of women ranging from perimenopausal to those already in menopause supplemented two scoops of herb maca into their diet daily. All participants experienced a reduction in menopausal symptoms. Tests also showed that their hormone levels were far more stable than before the study (Cabeca, n.d.).

Foods for Breaking Your Fast

When you break your fast, be wary of overindulging. Not only will you feel ill, but you will also be unable to spread out the rest of the meals you want to eat during your eating window and will likely end up much hungrier in your next fast. Always break your fast with a light meal that is easy to digest so that your sugar level rises relatively quickly, and then have your larger meal later in the day. By breaking your fast with a lighter meal, you will also soon be surprised at how easily your hunger is actually sated. You don't need an enormous plate of food to sustain you, even when you are fasting.

Hummus is an excellent option for breaking your fast. This dip (or spread) made from pureed chickpeas is delicious and satisfying. Eat it with cut up pieces of vegetables for a healthy meal to get you to dinner. Hummus also works well as a spread for crackers or rye bread.

Smoothies are another healthy fast-breaking meal. Pack your smoothies with as many vegetables and fruits as you can to increase your antioxidant and vitamin intake. Use frozen fruits and vegetables to make things easier for you—they have just as many vitamins as the fresh variety. Blueberries are one of the best ingredients for smoothies as they are packed with antioxidants.

Papaya contains papain, which helps to break down proteins more quickly. If you opt for a protein-dense snack to break your fast, include a few chunks of papaya to help release the protein into your system more quickly and aid digestion.

Break your fast with a handful of assorted nuts or eat them just before exercising to release an excellent source of protein into your body. Studies have also shown that people who eat nuts regularly have a lower risk of cardiovascular disease and Type 2 Diabetes (Weeks, 2019). Almonds and walnuts are particularly delicious when sprinkled over a salad or pasta dish. Peanut butter (preferably without added sugar) is a variation on nuts that is just as good for breaking your fast.

Avocado in a salad or on a piece of whole grain bread is a nice, light, yet nutritious way to break your fast. Avocado is a good source of unsaturated fat, and it is very filling. By adding just half an avocado to your lunch, you could feel fuller for several hours longer than if you hadn't eaten it. You could also slice up your avocado with a hard-boiled egg, which is a phenomenal source of protein and also keeps you fuller for longer.

Bone broths and vegetable soups are particularly good for breaking longer fasts but serve as a highly nutritious light meal for breaking any fast (Axe, 2019).

If you are breaking your fast when you are away from home, be sure that you are prepared. Pack your lunch at home the night before or ensure that you have a healthy option for bought food if that is necessary. Sandwiches are a nice light way to break your fast. Try and stick to whole wheat bread or wraps and include a protein source in your filling. Get yourself used to not using butter or margarine on your bread when your filling is saucy or moist. It just adds to the saturated fats that you are taking in and increases the calorie count as well. We tend to butter our bread out of habit, but if you are already eating a spread or a filling that has its own moisture, you don't even notice the butter.

The following are some ideas for healthy fillings to break your fast:

- **Egg salad:** Hard-boiled egg is a phenomenal source of protein. You can add a small amount of mayonnaise to it and some chopped tomato or cucumber.
- **Roast chicken and avocado:** This is a delightful combination of protein and unsaturated fat that will leave you feeling fuller for longer. If you make a roast chicken for dinner, keep some shredded chicken aside to enjoy this sandwich during the week.
- **Tuna salad:** Choose canned tuna in water to avoid the additional oil and finely chop some onion, tomato, and cucumber. The moisture from the tomato and cucumber means that you don't need any additional mayonnaise or other sauce, which just adds to the calories unnecessarily.

- **Steak:** Steak leftover from dinner the night before makes a great, satisfying filling for a sandwich with a scraping of mustard on the bread.
- **Roasted vegetables:** This is something that you can prepare a lot of at home and keep in the fridge for a few days to eat as sides or as fillings on sandwiches. Roast some peppers, tomatoes, onions, carrots and add some garlic and herbs to taste. This can be eaten cold on a sandwich with a slice of cheese as your protein.
- **Hummus:** This chickpea dish is as equally good on bread or wraps as it is when used as a dip. It is also highly nutritious and filling.
- **Pulled pork:** We all love our ham and cheese sandwiches, but processed meat is really unhealthy, and we are far better off preparing our own pork cut at home and shredding it to make a pulled pork sandwich. Pulled pork also goes really well with avocado and a sprinkling of fresh coriander.

Best Main Meal Options

Pasta has as bad a reputation as fat does, but for intermittent fasting, it is actually one of the best sustained-release sources of energy. As with anything, quality matters, and store-bought pasta is not the best option. Ideally, homemade pasta is your absolute best bet. If you aren't keen on making it yourself, you can buy handmade pasta at Italian delis and in some good health shops. By eating a good-sized serving of pasta as your final meal in your eating window, you maintain your blood sugar in a far more sustainable manner and stay fuller for longer. The great thing about pasta is that it is so versatile. You can mix your own combinations of toppings and sauces to your taste. Pack your sauce with vegetables, garlic, and a lean protein source to maximize your meal.

The ideal main meal consists of a serving of protein, including chicken, turkey, lamb, beef, lentils, or other legumes; two servings of vegetables (green leafy vegetables and cruciferous vegetables are ideal); and a carbohydrate, which includes potato, sweetcorn, or sweet potato. Your vegetable portion should always be at least twice the size of your protein and carbohydrate portions. If you stick to this formula and ensure that you are not eating more than you need to, you will maintain a healthy balance in nutrition. If you are eating a balanced diet, there is usually no need for additional supplements, but certain nutrients are difficult to get enough of from food and as we age, we do need more calcium, for instance, and rather than risking the possibility of developing brittle bones, get yourself onto a supplement for calcium.

A slow cooker or crockpot is a great tool when you are intermittent fasting as you can assemble your meal in the morning, including a lean form of protein and lots of vegetables, and then set it on low for the day. When you are ready to eat your main meal of the day during your eating window, you will have a healthy dinner prepared. The risk with intermittent fasting, if you are trying to lose weight, is that toward the end of your fast, your brain starts to tell you that you are really hungry. This, of course, is all in your head as you are likely not much hungrier at that point than during the rest of your fast, but your brain will tell you otherwise. This self-created desperation to eat could cause you to take in too many calories if you have not planned well. Always make sure that you have healthy snacks and low-calorie options available while you prepare your meal. You can have a few carrot sticks while you cook for instance. Planning is key here, as is realizing that what your brain is telling you is not always true.

You can also work on meal preparation when you have some downtime to make your life easier. If you are chopping two carrots and you have time, chop them all. Using frozen vegetables is usually just the same as using fresh from a nutrient standpoint, and it makes it far easier to keep an array of vegetables in the house if you don't have to worry about them spoiling.

As part of your weekly planning for fasting, you can also plan your meals to make your life even easier. That way you can also see at a glance whether you are getting in a balanced range of foodstuffs and all of the nutrients you need. Planning meals ahead of time also makes grocery shopping a lot easier, and you are far less likely to buy items that you don't need. Try not to do grocery shopping during your fasting window. It is a well-known fact that if we shop when we are hungry, we tend to buy far more than we need, and we also purchase far more junk food. Try and do your weekly grocery shopping either on a day when you are not fasting, which is ideal, or during your eating window after you have broken your fast with a light snack.

To sate a sweet tooth after dinner without ruining all your great progress on a giant plate of dessert, you can try a few squares of dark chocolate (no less than 60 percent cacao), which have a far lower impact on blood sugar than other sweets (Ball, n.d.). Fruit is also great for satisfying a need for something sweet, so your berry smoothies work brilliantly for breaking your fast and as a dessert.

Fasting-Friendly Recipes - Light Meals

The following recipes have been chosen to align with the suggestions we have made for breaking fasts in the previous section. These specific foods have been selected for their ability to provide a lift to blood sugar levels and also to sustain those levels throughout the day. If you have other foods you would like to try, you can look up the nutritional references online quite easily and fit them into your fasting plan.

Hello Hummus!

The debate about whether to use canned chickpeas or chickpeas soaked overnight in making hummus has been raging since...well since canned chickpeas were invented! Most say that the negligible difference in taste is really not worth the hassle and the nutritional content is exactly the same.

Nutritional Information (per serving):

- Carbohydrates   12.4 g
- Protein   7.5 g
- Fat   5.1 g
- Fiber   2.6 g
- Salt   0.5 g
- Calories   135

Time: 5 minutes

Special Equipment: Food processor

Serving Size: ¼ of total yield

Ingredients:

- 1 x 14-ounce can of chickpeas
- 1 large chopped garlic clove
- 1 tbsp tahini paste
- A squeeze of lemon juice

- 3 tbsps Greek yogurt

Directions:

1. Drain chickpeas through a sieve over a jug to catch the liquid. Set liquid aside.
2. In a food processor, place chickpeas, tahini paste, lemon juice, and Greek yogurt and process until smooth.
3. Add a tablespoon of the chickpea liquid at a time, running the food processor after each addition, until you reach your desired consistency.
4. For a dip, you may want a slightly looser consistency, while a hummus spread will need to be a little thicker.

Suggestions & Variations:

If you would like a sweeter, more pungent garlic flavor, roast your clove of garlic before adding to your mix. Roasted red bell peppers also make an interesting addition to hummus.

Slimming Smoothie

The oats in this smoothie allow for sustained blood sugar for a longer period so that you feel fuller for longer.

Nutritional Information (per serving):

- Carbohydrates   56 g
- Protein   13 g
- Fat   2 g
- Fiber   6 g
- Salt   0 g
- Calories   280

Time: 5 minutes

Special Equipment: Blender

Serving Size: 1 smoothie (total yield)

Ingredients:

- ½ banana
- 1 cup strawberry slices
- ¼ cup rolled oats
- 1 cup milk
- ¼ tsp vanilla extract
- ½ cup ice chips
- 1 tsp honey

Directions:

1. In a blender, add your banana, strawberries, oats, and milk.
2. Blend until all the ingredients reach a smooth consistency.

3. Add the vanilla, ice chips, and honey and blend again until all the ingredients are completely mixed.
4. If you prefer a thinner consistency, add a little more milk or water and blend again after each addition.

Suggestions & Variations:

Don't peel your banana before cutting. That way, you can keep your second banana half for another smoothie without it going brown.

Very Veggie Smoothie

The rich green color of this smoothie makes it an exciting way to break your fast. It is also high in fiber to ensure the rest of your day is regular and comfortable.

Nutritional Information (per serving):

- Carbohydrates   27 g
- Protein   7 g
- Fat   10 g
- Fiber   6 g
- Salt   0.4 g
- Calories   243

Time: 5 minutes

Special Equipment: Blender

Serving Size: 1 smoothie (total yield)

Ingredients:

- 2 celery sticks
- 2 oz chopped spinach
- 3.5 oz broccoli florets
- 1 banana
- 1 cup of rice milk
- ¼ tsp spirulina
- 4 tbsps coconut
- 1 cup water

Directions:

1. In a blender, add spinach, celery, and broccoli.
2. Blend until all the vegetables reach a smooth consistency.
3. Add the banana, spirulina, coconut, rice milk, and water and blend again until all the ingredients are completely mixed.
4. If you prefer a thinner consistency, add a little more milk or water and blend again after each addition.

Suggestions & Variations:

The spirulina can be swapped out for vegan protein powder if you prefer.

Perfectly Papaya Salad

The papaya in this delicious salad helps you to quickly digest the protein available in the peanuts, leaving you quickly satisfied.

Nutritional Information (per serving):

- Carbohydrates   21 g
- Protein   10 g
- Fat   7 g
- Fiber   7 g
- Salt   0.1 g
- Calories   198

Time: 15 minutes

Special Equipment: None

Serving Size: ½ total yield

Ingredients:

- 1 cubed papaya
- 6 oz snow peas
- 6 oz bean sprouts
- A handful of unsalted peanuts
- Chopped fresh basil

- Chopped fresh mint
- Juice of 1 lime

Directions:

1. In a large frying pan, heat on high, add the snow peas and bean sprouts as well as one tablespoon of water.
2. Allow to stir fry for 3 minutes or until just tender.
3. Remove the snow peas and bean sprouts from the heat and transfer to a large salad bowl.
4. Add the papaya and lime juice and toss well.
5. Scatter the basil, mint, and peanuts over the top of the salad and serve immediately.

Suggestions & Variations:

Salads like this open themselves up for lots of creative interpretation. Swap your peanuts out for walnuts for a higher protein boost or use different herbs over the top depending on your taste.

Fruit & Nut Delight

The oats in this dish sustain your blood sugar levels for a longer period, while the nuts provide you with your protein and also assist in leaving you feeling fuller for longer.

Nutritional Information (per serving):

- Carbohydrates   35 g
- Protein   15 g
- Fat   11 g
- Fiber   7 g
- Salt   0.1 g
- Calories   316

Time: 10 minutes

Special Equipment: Nonstick pan

Serving Size: ½ total yield

Ingredients:

- 2 oz mixed raisins, seeds, nuts, and goji berries
- 6 tbsps oats
- 2 oranges
- 3.5 oz Greek yogurt
- 1 ¾ cup water

Directions:

1. Cut, peel, and chop the oranges and set aside.
2. Cook oats with water in a nonstick pan for about 4 minutes or until cooked and thickened.
3. Divide the oats into two breakfast bowls, spoon the yogurt over the top, and scatter the chopped oranges, nuts, raisins, seeds, and goji berries over the top.

Suggestions & Variations:

Swap the oranges out for a fruit that is in season or one that you prefer.

Avocado Bread Salad

This dish has the unsaturated fats from the avocado and the boost of carbs from the bread to keep you going until your next meal. The tomatoes are an excellent source of antioxidants.

Nutritional Information (per serving):

- Carbohydrates   30 g
- Protein   7 g

- Fat — 21 g
- Fiber — 6 g
- Salt — 0.9 g
- Calories — 332

Time: 20 minutes

Special Equipment: None

Serving Size: ¼ total yield

Ingredients:

- 1 ripe avocado
- 6 oz ciabatta or French loaf
- 28 oz ripe cherry tomatoes
- 1 crushed garlic clove
- 1 ½ tbsp capers
- 1 small, sliced red onion
- A handful of chopped, fresh basil
- 2 tbsps red wine vinegar
- 4 tbsps extra-virgin olive oil
- Seasoning to taste

Directions:

1. Halve the cherry tomatoes and place in a bowl. Season to taste and add avocado, onion, capers, and garlic. Mix well and allow to stand for 10 minutes;

this gives all of the flavors the opportunity to infuse into one another.

2. Slice the ciabatta or French loaf into approximately 1-inch pieces and arrange on a platter. Drizzle the bread with half of the extra-virgin olive oil and half of the red wine vinegar. Season to taste.

3. Pour the tomato mixture over the ciabatta or French loaf and mix gently. Scatter the basil leaves over the top and pour the remaining extra-virgin olive oil and red wine vinegar over the salad. Serve immediately.

Suggestions & Variations:

Cherry tomatoes are not an absolute necessity for this dish. You can use normal salad tomatoes as well and just chop them up into relatively small pieces.

Slow-Cooked Bone Broth

This bone broth can be made overnight in a slow cooker or crockpot. Slow cooking is essential for bone broths as it slowly draws the plethora of vitamins, nutrients, and minerals out of the bones without destroying any. The recipe yields four servings, which you can keep in the fridge or freeze for other fasting days. The longer you cook the broth, the darker it becomes. If you have pets, this bone broth is great for them as well!

Nutritional Information (per serving):

- Carbohydrates   4 g
- Protein   6 g
- Fat   0.3 g
- Fiber   0.2 g
- Salt   0.65 g
- Calories   45

Time: 18 - 36 hours

Special Equipment: Slow cooker or crockpot

Serving Size: ¼ total yield

Ingredients:

- Chicken, veal, or beef bones
- 1 celery stick
- 2 chopped carrots
- 1 leek
- 1 bay leaf
- Juice of 1 lemon
- Water to fill slow cooker

Directions:

1. Preheat the oven to 350°F.
2. On a baking tray, scatter the bones and roast for one hour. Turn them over halfway through the time.
3. In the meantime, peel and chop your vegetables and place into the slow cooker with the bay leaf and lemon juice.
4. When your bones are roasted, remove from the baking sheet and place on top of your vegetables in the slow cooker.
5. Fill with water until about ½ an inch from the top. Cover and cook on low for 18 - 36 hours.
6. After cooking, place a sieve over a bowl and scoop the bones into the sieve. Once all of the bones are out of your broth, return any broth that has collected in the bowl to the slow cooker.
7. Strain all of the contents of the slow cooker (in batches if need be) to remove any solid pieces. Add additional seasoning if required.
8. Allow to cool and remove any fat that has surfaced on the top.

Suggestions & Variations:

Use relatively large bones for this recipe to make the removal process easier.

Veggie Soup

The potato and root vegetables in this brightly colored dish provide sustained energy until your next meal and are also packed with nutrients.

Nutritional Information (per serving):

- Carbohydrates   16 g
- Protein   7 g
- Fat   4 g
- Fiber   0.2 g
- Salt   0.5 g
- Calories   127

Time: 25 minutes

Special Equipment: None

Serving Size: ⅙ total yield

Ingredients:

- 1 large potato
- 1 bunch of green onions

- 4 oz spinach
- 9 oz frozen peas
- 4 ¼ cup vegetable stock
- 1 ¼ cup plain yogurt
- 1 crushed garlic clove
- Mint, basil, or cress leaves to serve

Directions:

1. In a large pot, bring vegetable stock, potato, and garlic to a boil.
2. Once boiling, reduce to a simmer, cover with a lid, and allow to cook for 15 minutes or until the potato is soft.
3. Add the frozen peas to the pot and allow to simmer again. Remove about four tablespoons of peas from the pot and set aside to use as garnish later.
4. Remove from heat and stir in spinach and yogurt.
5. Blend soup mixture with a stick blender until very smooth and season to taste.
6. After dishing into bowls, sprinkle with the peas you set aside and the fresh herbs of your choice.

Suggestions & Variations:

This soup is deliciously satisfying as is, but if you would like an extra boost of carbohydrates, you can enjoy it with a slice of crusty bread.

BBQ Beef Salad

The potato and root vegetables in this brightly colored dish provide sustained energy until your next meal and are also packed with nutrients.

Nutritional Information (per serving):

- Carbohydrates   7 g
- Protein   21 g
- Fat   17 g
- Fiber   6 g
- Salt   0.4 g
- Calories   281

Time: 25 minutes (plus one hour to rest)

Special Equipment: Barbeque

Serving Size: ⅙ total yield

Ingredients:

- 2 x 9 oz sirloin steaks
- 2 tbsp sesame oil

- 1 tbsp low-sodium soy sauce
- 1 sliced chili
- 2 finely chopped chilies
- ½-inch piece of ginger, grated
- 1 clove of garlic
- The juice of 2 limes
- 4 baby heads of lettuce
- 12 radishes
- 3 spring onions
- 1 large ripe avocado
- ½ tbsp sesame seeds
- 3 carrots
- ½ cucumber

Directions:

1. Ensure that you remove the steak from the fridge at least an hour before you plan to start cooking so that it reaches room temperature.
2. To prepare your salad dressing, combine the garlic, lime juice, ginger, oil, soy sauce, and chopped chilies and set aside.
3. Cook the steaks on the barbeque for 3 minutes per side until medium-rare. Rest for 5 minutes after cooking and before slicing.

4. Chop and slice the lettuces, radishes, carrots, spring onions, avocado, and cucumber and arrange on a platter.
5. Slice the steak and spread over the top of the vegetables.
6. Drizzle with the dressing and garnish with sesame seeds and chili.
7. Serve immediately.

Suggestions & Variations:

The flavor of barbequed meat is just tastier in this salad, but if you don't have access to one, you can fry in a griddle pan as well.

Fasting-Friendly Main Meal Recipes

The key to preparing main meals that work well with fasting is ensuring that your energy is sustained until you break your fast the next day. Your metabolism will slow down while you sleep, so you shouldn't eat your main meal any less than 2 hours before you plan to go to sleep. The recipes we have chosen to share with you here are family-friendly recipes that you can enjoy at the dinner table with your loved ones. They have the added benefit of being fasting friendly too.

Salmon Pasta

Pasta is a fantastic slow-release energy source. Paired with wild-caught salmon, this dish is brain food and a healthy source of protein too. It has a high-fat content, but these are unsaturated (good) fats from the salmon.

Nutritional Information (per serving):

- Carbohydrates 77 g
- Protein 42 g
- Fat 25 g
- Fiber 4 g
- Salt 0.21 g
- Calories 682

Time: 25 minutes

Special Equipment: Nonstick pan

Serving Size: ½ total yield

Ingredients:

- 7 oz tagliatelle pasta
- 2 wild-caught salmon fillets
- 3.5 oz rocket
- 2 tbsps creme fraiche
- 1 tsp extra-virgin olive oil
- Zest of 1 lemon

Directions:

1. Heat a large nonstick skillet over high heat with one teaspoon of extra-virgin olive oil. Place the salmon fillets skin-side down into the pan and fry for 5 minutes on one side, then turn and fry for another 4 minutes on the other side.
2. Remove the salmon fillets from the pan, allow to cool, and remove the skin. Flake into large chunks and set aside.
3. In a pot, cook the pasta until al dente. Reserve one cup of the cooking water, drain the pasta, and return to the pot.
4. Add the salmon chunks, rocket, creme fraiche, and lemon zest to pasta and use the cup of reserved cooking water to loosen the mixture. Stir well, taking care not to mash up the salmon pieces.

Suggestions & Variations:

Tagliatelle works best with this dish, but you can use any pasta of your choice.

Chicken Balti

Poultry is one of the best sources of animal protein. By removing the skin, you can further reduce the fat content.

Nutritional Information (per serving):

- Carbohydrates   31 g
- Protein   40 g
- Fat   6 g
- Fiber   9 g
- Salt   0.6 g
- Calories   341

Time: 60 minutes

Special Equipment: Large, deep nonstick pan

Serving Size: ½ total yield

Ingredients:

- 4 boned and skinned chicken thighs
- 1 onion
- 1 yellow pepper
- 1 red pepper

- 2 garlic cloves
- 8 oz canned tomatoes
- 3 tbsps chopped cilantro
- Additional cilantro for garnish
- ⅔ cup plain yogurt
- 1 tbsp curry powder
- 1 tbsp cornflour
- Black pepper
- Extra-virgin olive oil for frying
- 2 tbsps cold water
- 3 ½ oz water

Directions:

1. Heat oil in a large, nonstick frying pan over medium heat and add chopped onion. Allow onion to fry until translucent.
2. Trim any visible fat off the chicken pieces and cut each thigh into quarters. Season with black pepper.
3. Add the peppers and chicken pieces into the pan with the onion and allow to cook for 3 minutes, turning the chicken pieces occasionally.
4. In a small bowl, mix the cornflour with the two tablespoons of water and add the yogurt. Mix well.

5. Add the garlic and curry powder to the pan with the chicken and cook for 30 seconds.

6. Add the yogurt mixture, three-and-a-half ounces of water, cilantro, and canned tomatoes to the pan and bring to a simmer. Cook for 25 minutes until chicken is cooked through and the sauce has thickened.

7. Season with black pepper and sprinkle the cilantro garnish over the top.

Suggestions & Variations:

This recipe also works with turkey. Serve as is or with your choice of carbohydrate.

Meatless Spaghetti Bolognaise

This vegetarian dish is packed with healthy plant-based protein.

Nutritional Information (per serving):

- Carbohydrates   61 g
- Protein   19 g
- Fat   15 g
- Fiber   19 g

- Salt   0.4 g
- Calories   494

Time: 45 minutes

Special Equipment: None

Serving Size: ¼ total yield

Ingredients:

- 15 oz canned lentils
- 8 oz cooked whole grain spaghetti
- 1 oz dehydrated porcini mushrooms
- 1 chopped onion
- 1 chopped carrot
- 1 leek
- 1 stick of celery
- 2 cloves of garlic
- ¼ cup of extra-virgin olive oil
- Salt and pepper for seasoning
- 1 bay leaf
- ½ tsp dried oregano
- ½ tsp dried basil
- ½ tsp dried thyme
- ¼ cup almond milk
- 15 oz canned tomatoes with juice
- 2 tbsps tomato paste
- Shaved parmesan for garnish

Directions:

1. Soak dehydrated porcini mushrooms in warm water for 15 minutes. Remove mushrooms when rehydrated and pat dry on a paper towel. Chop mushrooms finely.
2. Chop celery, leek, carrot, onion, and garlic and mix together.
3. Heat oil in a large pan over medium heat and add onion mixture and mushrooms to the pan and cook for 8 minutes or until the vegetables are soft.
4. Add almond milk, bay leaf, herbs, and lentils and cook for about 3 minutes, stirring occasionally.
5. When the liquid in the pan has almost completely evaporated, add the can of tomatoes and the paste.
6. Mix well and continue cooking for another 10 minutes, stirring frequently to avoid scorching.
7. Remove the bay leaf and serve on top of a bed of pasta.

Suggestions & Variations:

Serve with a slice of garlic bread or a small side salad.

Saucy Steaks with Sweet Potato Fries

While you don't want to overdo red meat, if it's something you enjoy occasionally, that's just fine. The key is to keep your portion small and serve with healthy sides.

Nutritional Information (per serving):

- Carbohydrates   43 g
- Protein   33 g
- Fat   0.5 g
- Fiber   12 g
- Salt   0.4 g
- Calories   452

Time: 35 minutes

Special Equipment: None

Serving Size: ½ total yield

Ingredients:

- 2 x 4.5 oz fillet steaks
- 9 oz sweet potato
- 7 oz baby spinach
- 2 onions
- 1 green pepper
- 3 oz cherry tomatoes
- 3 tbsps extra-virgin olive oil

- 1 tbsp fresh thyme
- 1 tsp paprika
- 2 cloves of garlic
- 1 tbsp tomato paste
- 1 tbsp vegetable bouillon powder
- 5 oz water

Directions:

1. Preheat the oven to 475°F.
2. Peel your sweet potato and slice into thin fries. Place in a bowl with two tablespoons of the oil and the thyme. Toss to coat the fries.
3. Scatter the sweet potato fries on a wire rack and place the rack over a baking tray to catch dripping oil. Set aside for now.
4. Heat up a nonstick pan with one teaspoon of oil. Add the onions, cover, and allow to cook until translucent (about 5 minutes). Add the green pepper and garlic and cook for another 5 minutes.
5. Put your sweet potato fries into the oven and bake for 15 minutes.
6. Stir the paprika and water into the pan with your onion mixture and add the tomato paste, bouillon powder, and

cherry tomatoes. Simmer with the lid on for 10 minutes.

7. Rub your steaks with a little extra-virgin olive oil. Pan fry for about 3 minutes on each side depending on how thick your steaks are. Allow to rest for 5 minutes.
8. Wilt your spinach quickly in a pan or in the microwave.
9. Plate up and spoon the sauce over the steaks with your wilted spinach and sweet potato fries on the side.

Suggestions & Variations:

If you prefer another cut of steak, that is your choice, but keep it as lean as possible to keep those saturated fats down.

Mexican Pasta

You will likely only need a small portion of this pasta to fill you up as both the pasta and the avocado are great for sustained energy release.

Nutritional Information (per serving):

- Carbohydrates   65 g
- Protein   15 g

- Fat   15 g
- Fiber   18 g
- Salt   0.4 g
- Calories   495

Time: 30 minutes

Special Equipment: None

Serving Size: ½ total yield

Ingredients:

- 3.5 oz whole wheat penne
- 1 large avocado
- 1 onion
- 2 cloves of garlic
- 1 yellow pepper
- 14 oz canned tomatoes
- 7 oz canned corn kernels
- Zest and juice of half a lime
- 1 tsp vegetable bouillon powder
- Handful of cilantro
- Additional cilantro to garnish
- 1 tsp extra-virgin olive oil
- 2 tsps ground chili
- ½ tsp cumin seeds
- 1 tsp ground cilantro
- 1 tbsp finely chopped onion

Directions:

1. Cook the pasta until al dente.
2. Heat a pan with oil over medium heat and fry the pepper and onion while stirring until translucent. Add the garlic, tomatoes, spices, bouillon, corn, and half of the water in which corn is canned.
3. Simmer for 15 minutes.
4. Drizzle the avocado with the lime juice and toss together with the finely chopped onion.
5. Drain the penne and stir into the sauce, adding the cilantro.
6. Plate up the pasta, spoon avocado mixture over it, and garnish with cilantro.

Suggestions & Variations:

If you prefer this a little spicier, add some fresh finely chopped chili to the avocado mix.

Spicy Chickpea and Lentil Soup

Both the chickpeas and lentils in this delicious, chunky soup are excellent sources of sustained energy and will keep you feeling full for longer. This soup freezes very well, so you can make a pot and freeze the rest to ensure you have lunches and dinners at hand in the future.

Nutritional Information (per serving):

- Carbohydrates   17.2 g
- Protein   8.5 g
- Fat   2.4 g
- Fiber   6.1 g
- Salt   0.4 g
- Calories   136

Time: 40 minutes

Special Equipment: Electric Pressure Cooker

Serving Size: 1 cup

Ingredients:

- 1 cup lentils
- 1 cup dried chickpeas (soaked overnight)
- 1 onion
- 2 celery stalks
- 14 oz canned tomatoes
- 3 cups chicken stock
- 2 tbsps lime juice
- 15 oz chopped pumpkin

- ½ tsp dried chili
- 3 cups water
- ½ cup chopped cilantro
- 2 tsps extra-virgin olive oil
- 3 cloves of garlic
- 2 tsps paprika
- 1 ½ inch piece of fresh ginger
- 1 tsp ground cumin
- 1 tsp ground cilantro

Directions:

1. Drain your chickpeas that have soaked overnight and rinse with cold water.
2. In a 24-cup pressure cooker, heat oil and then cook onion, garlic, and grated ginger until the onion softens.
3. Add the ground cilantro, ground cumin, paprika, and dried chili and cook until fragrant.
4. Add the water, stock, tomatoes, and chickpeas. Secure the lid of your pressure cooker and set to high pressure for 25 minutes.
5. Release pressure after 25 minutes have passed and carefully remove the lid, pointing the steam away from your face.

6. Add the lentils, pumpkin, and celery and secure the lid again.
7. Bring to high pressure and cook for 5 minutes. Release pressure and set to simmer for another 5 minutes. Stir in lime juice and fresh cilantro.

Suggestions & Variations:

If you don't have a pressure cooker, this soup can be made in a slow cooker and on the stovetop as well. Cook until the chickpeas and lentils are soft. This is intended to be a chunky soup, and it is not necessary to liquidize it.

Lamb Navarin

Lamb is one of the healthier red meats and can be enjoyed in stews and curries.

Nutritional Information (per serving):

- Carbohydrates — 31.2 g
- Protein — 34 g
- Fat — 21.9 g
- Fiber — 9.6 g
- Salt — 0.4 g
- Calories — 477

Time: 95 minutes

Special Equipment: None

Serving Size: ¼ of total yield

Ingredients:

- 4 lamb neck chops
- 1 onion
- 2 cloves of garlic
- 14 oz canned tomatoes
- ½ cup water
- 8 baby onions
- 12 ½ oz baby carrots
- 1 cup frozen peas
- 2 tbsps fresh flat-leaf parsley
- 1 tbsp extra-virgin olive oil
- 1 pound baby potatoes

Directions:

1. Heat a large pot over medium heat with extra-virgin olive oil. Brown lamb in batches. The key to browning is that the more color you are able to get on your lamb, the more flavor you will have. You don't want to burn the meat, of course, but this process also helps to break down the fat in the lamb.

2. When your lamb is browned, remove
    from the pot and cook the chopped
    onion and garlic until the onion is
    translucent. Add your lamb back into
    the pot with the tomatoes and water.
    Bring to boil and then allow to cook for
    30 - 45 minutes with the lid on. Stir
    occasionally to avoid sticking on the
    bottom of the pot. This process softens
    the meat without destroying any of the
    other ingredients.
3. When your meat has started to soften,
    stir in the potatoes and baby onions
    and sprinkle the carrots over the top.
    Allow to cook for 15 minutes or until
    the potatoes and carrots are soft.
4. Add peas and allow to simmer until
    peas are tender and warmed through.
    Season to taste and sprinkle with
    parsley when serving.

Suggestions & Variations:

Lamb takes time to soften, so this isn't a dish
that can be done in a casserole form as the
remaining ingredients will be too soft and the
meat will still be tough. The fat on lamb is one
of the healthier forms of animal fat, but in a
dish like this, it is preferable to reduce the

amount of fat by trimming away as much as possible before cooking.

Chili Braised Pork

This low carbohydrate and high protein meal is great for those who are trying to lose weight or muscle training.

Nutritional Information (per serving):

- Carbohydrates 8.1 g
- Protein 44.6 g
- Fat 26 g
- Fiber 2 g
- Salt 0.5 g
- Calories 447

Time: 60 minutes

Special Equipment: Kitchen string

Serving Size: ¼ of total yield

Ingredients:

- 1 ½ pounds boned pork shoulder
- 4 cloves of garlic
- 4 anchovy fillets
- 14 oz canned tomatoes
- 1 cup of water

- 2 tbsps extra-virgin olive oil
- 2 tbsps fresh oregano
- 1 tbsp capers
- ½ tsp dried chili
- ½ cup black seeded olives

Directions:

1. Roll the pork shoulder and tie with kitchen string at ¾ -inch intervals to hold the meat together.
2. Heat a large pan and brown your pork shoulder to seal the meat and retain the juices while cooking. When browned, remove from the pan and set aside.
3. Heat oil in the pot and cook garlic and anchovy, stirring until fragrant. Stir in the tomatoes, water, oregano, chili, and capers. Return the pork to the pot and cook for 40 minutes. When the pork is still slightly pink but tender, remove from the pot. If you prefer your pork cooked more, you can keep it cooking for another 5 minutes or so. After removing, allow to stand for 5 minutes before removing the string and slicing. This allows the fibers in the meat to

stick together so that the meat slices more cleanly.

4. Stir the olives into the sauce and season to taste. Serve slices of the pork shoulder on a bed of creamy polenta and covered in the sauce.

Suggestions & Variations:

Instead of polenta, you can also serve this dish with a slice of crusty bread to mop up the sauce.

Butter Chicken

One of the most popular mild dishes of Indian origin, butter chicken is a perfect meal for the whole family, and its use of lean protein makes it healthy as well.

Nutritional Information (per serving):

- Carbohydrates   23.5 g
- Protein   48.7 g
- Fat   58.1 g
- Fiber   4 g
- Salt   0.5 g
- Calories   814

Time: 60 minutes

Special Equipment: None

Serving Size: ¼ of total yield

Ingredients:

- 4 chicken breasts
- 1 tbsp lemon juice
- ½ cup plain yogurt
- 2-inch piece of ginger, grated
- 2 tsp garam masala
- 1 tbsp vegetable oil
- 1 ½ oz butter
- 1 onion
- 4 cloves of garlic
- 1 tsp ground cilantro
- 1 tsp ground cumin
- 1 tsp ground cinnamon
- 1 tsp paprika
- 2 tbsps tomato paste
- 14 oz canned tomato puree
- ½ chicken stock
- 2 tbsps honey
- ⅓ cup pouring cream
- ½ cup fresh cilantro

Directions:

1. Mix chicken, lemon juice, ginger, yogurt, and garam masala in a large

bowl. Ensure the chicken is well coated in the marinade.

2. In a large, heavy-bottomed pot, heat half of the oil and half of the butter and brown the marinated chicken in batches. Remove from the pot and set aside.
3. Heat the remaining oil and butter in the pot and cook the onion and garlic until the onion is soft.
4. Return the chicken to the pot with the tomato paste, tomato puree, chicken stock, and honey. Cook for 30 minutes or until chicken is tender and cooked through.
5. Stir in the cream and season to taste.
6. Plate up and serve garnished with fresh cilantro.

Suggestions & Variations:

Serve with your choice of starch. You can increase the strength of this dish by adding more garam masala if you wish.

Conclusion

As women over 50, we are forewarned to expect health challenges as we get older. We see our friends and family members experiencing weight gain, menopausal symptoms, and the onset of noncommunicable diseases such as diabetes and hypertension. We enter this time in our lives with a sense of trepidation, feeling out of control and like our bodies are working against us. The reality could not be further from the truth. There are certainly specific health concerns that we need to look out for, but our 50s and above could actually be the time in our lives when we have the most vitality as we are no longer focusing our energies on others, and we have more time to support our own needs and goals. This should actually be an exciting time for us, and if we learn the right tools and educate ourselves on what is really happening in our bodies, it can be.

As we enter our 50s, there is no greater opportunity to get our physical and mental health where we want it to be. We are at a stage in our lives where we can focus our attention on taking care of ourselves.

Intermittent fasting is one of the most holistic methods of doing this. Through a very simple practice of structuring the way we eat, we can offset the effects of aging, lose weight, reduce and sometimes completely eliminate certain diseases, and increase our longevity. Through intermittent fasting, rather than feeling like our body is working against us, we are actually using our body's natural processes to our advantage. We have far greater control over our bodies than we like to think we do. The key is to harness the way our body works, and in order to do that, we need to understand it. At this age, many of us have engaged in dieting and have come to realize that fad diets do us more harm than good.

The flexibility of intermittent fasting means that we can structure it around our lifestyles and not vise versa. Most weight loss programs fail because they are too difficult to keep up with or because the food items you need to eat are too expensive. Fasting doesn't dictate what to eat, and you choose when to eat. As long as you maintain an overall healthy diet, you can indulge in your favorite food occasionally without feeling like you are letting yourself down. It is this very flexibility and the idea that you are not 'punishing' yourself that makes intermittent fasting probably the easiest weight loss regime to follow.

When you first start intermittent fasting and explain to others what you are doing, you can be prepared for a few frowns and points of misunderstanding. People generally see fasting as something strange, and they may wonder why you are putting yourself through such a 'terrible' thing. You can handle this in one of two ways. You can either explain to them what you have learned in this book so that they too understand intermittent fasting, or you can smile and tell them that they shouldn't worry about you because you will be just fine. The former would, of course, be more helpful to them as they may even try fasting after hearing you explain it, but not everyone is able to open their mind enough to accept that what they have been taught about food for years is largely incorrect. Suffice to say that when they see the results you are getting, they will probably be more open to considering fasting.

Fasting is an age-old practice. If the fad diets presenting themselves in the last few years make you skeptical, you are not alone. Many of these fashionable diets have very little basis in science. They have also only been practiced for a few years, so there is really very little long-term evidence of their effects on our bodies. While this may not be too much of an issue for someone in their early 20s, as we get older, we need to make sure that what we are undertaking with our health has scientific backing. Thankfully, intermittent fasting has significant clinical research as well as real-life results backing up the purported benefits. Fasting works with the processes in our bodies that are already there; it just enhances them and stabilizes them.

Fasting doesn't just help us with weight loss either; it has benefits throughout our body and even cognitively as well as emotionally. While there are some slight effects in the first few days of fasting, none of these are insurmountable, and with some planning and preparation, you can work through them easily. The side effects last a very short period, and your body easily adjusts to what is essentially its natural process.

Our bodies are actually not made to eat constantly, and from an evolutionary perspective, we are far more aligned to a fasting regime than constant feeding. This is proven by the fact that so many beneficial processes occur naturally in our bodies when we fast. Food is important from the perspective of taking in nutrients, and it is also enjoyable to eat, but our society has turned food into our enemy rather than our friend.

If you consider the fact that just 20 years ago, the World Health Organization's biggest focus and challenge was undernutrition and starvation and as of 2019, their main focus is now obesity and overnutrition, this displays exactly how badly we have skewed our relationship with food. The World Health Organization has even coined a term for the way we now eat; it is called the "Westernized Diet." The term is not complimentary either as it denotes a way of eating that focuses mainly on convenience foods, high levels of sugar, and a large consumption of red meat.

This "Westernized Diet" is not just a problem in the US. As advertising spreads across the world, it is becoming popularized in many countries, and studies are showing a significant negative shift in countries where the overall diet used to be healthy.

Alcohol has also become a huge problem for health, and many women over 50 struggle with belly fat due to high sugar alcoholic drinks. While alcohol does not need to be avoided completely, it should certainly be minimized, especially as we age, and it has a greater impact on our bodies.

Overnutrition is just as dangerous as undernutrition, and it is one of the leading risk factors for most noncommunicable diseases. As we age, we have the opportunity to start caring for our bodies in a way we may not have in the past. Keep in mind that you do not need to change your entire family's lifestyle in order to change your own. Fasting fits in well with our lives as they are, so it's not necessary for anyone else in your household to make changes. By fasting, you are not only ensuring a better life for yourself but also for your family. You will have more energy, live longer, and have a better quality of life when spending time with your loved ones. That alone is worth working for.

A healthy diet overall includes plenty of fresh fruit and vegetables, lean protein (preferably plant-based or very lean animal protein), unsaturated fats, and plenty of fiber. Processed foods with high sodium and saturated fat levels are a no-no in any eating plan. Including plenty of fresh fruit and vegetables in your eating window also ups your level of antioxidants, and when this is paired with the natural fasting benefit of autophagy, it has additional benefits for a longer lifespan.

In *Intermittent Fasting For Women over 50*, we have given you all of the information you need in order to make fasting part of your lifestyle. Our food suggestions can be adjusted to your own preferences, as can the recipes we have supplied. By using the general food ideas that we have given you, you can also seek out further resources to find new recipes. In food choices, balance is key. It is not necessary to deny yourself something that you really enjoy just because it may contain a few calories. As much as food is about supporting our body's processes, it is also about enjoyment, and there's really no need for us to restrict ourselves so severely that we feel as though we are merely existing and not enjoying life.

It cannot be denied that when we socialize, food is a big part of that enjoyment, and that is not a bad thing. As long as we do not overdo our eating or use festivities as an excuse to binge, then there is no problem with associating socializing with food. Fasting should add to your life and never detract from it, so if you are finding it punishing or something that you dread doing after a few months of consistent fasting, then you may want to look at how you are fasting. Often, with just a small change such as slightly shortening our fasting time or changing the times at which we fast, we can completely switch our experience of intermittent fasting. The idea is to reach your weight goals while also enjoying extra energy, increased vitality, and overall wellness.

Entering your 50s needn't be a time of difficulty or trepidation, and the intermittent fasting lifestyle is key to ensuring you are living your best life from all perspectives.

References

6 Popular Ways to Do Intermittent Fasting. (2017). Healthline. https://www.healthline.com/nutrition/6-ways-to-do-intermittent-fasting

11 High-Energy Foods for Intermittent Fasting. (n.d.). Food Network. Retrieved February 21, 2020, from https://www.foodnetwork.com/healthyeats/diets/2019/07/high-energy-foods-intermittent-fasting

Fung, J. (2019, April 25). Diet Doctor. Diet Doctor. https://www.dietdoctor.com/intermittent-fasting

Gunnars, K. (2017, June 4). What Is Intermittent Fasting? Explained in Human Terms. Healthline; Healthline Media. https://www.healthline.com/nutrition/what-is-intermittent-fasting#section2

How Intermittent Fasting and a Healthy Diet Boost Mental Health. (2019, May 1). 24Life. https://www.24life.com/how-intermittent-fasting-and-a-healthy-diet-boost-mental-health/

I Went Into Early Perimenopause & Learned Why Balancing Blood Sugar Is So Important. (2019, January 30). Mindbodygreen. https://www.mindbodygreen.com/articles/blood-sugar-and-perimenopause

Jeanie Lerche Davis. (2007, March 23). Get-Fit Advice for Women Over 50. WebMD; WebMD. https://www.webmd.com/women/guide/women-over-50-fitness-tips

Kresser, C. (2019, March 25). Intermittent Fasting: The Science Behind the Trend. Chris Kresser; chriskresser.com. https://chriskresser.com/intermittent-fasting-the-science-behind-the-trend/

Pawlowski, A. (2019, January 16). How to lose weight with intermittent fasting, 16:8 diet. TODAY.Com; TODAY. https://www.today.com/health/how-lose-weight-intermittent-fasting-16-8-diet-t132608

Practical tips for fasting. (2016, September 15). Diet Doctor. https://www.dietdoctor.com/practical-tips-fasting

What Foods Are Best to Eat on an Intermittent Fasting Diet? (n.d.). Greatist. Retrieved February 21, 2020, from https://greatist.com/eat/what-to-eat-on-an-intermittent-fasting-diet#1

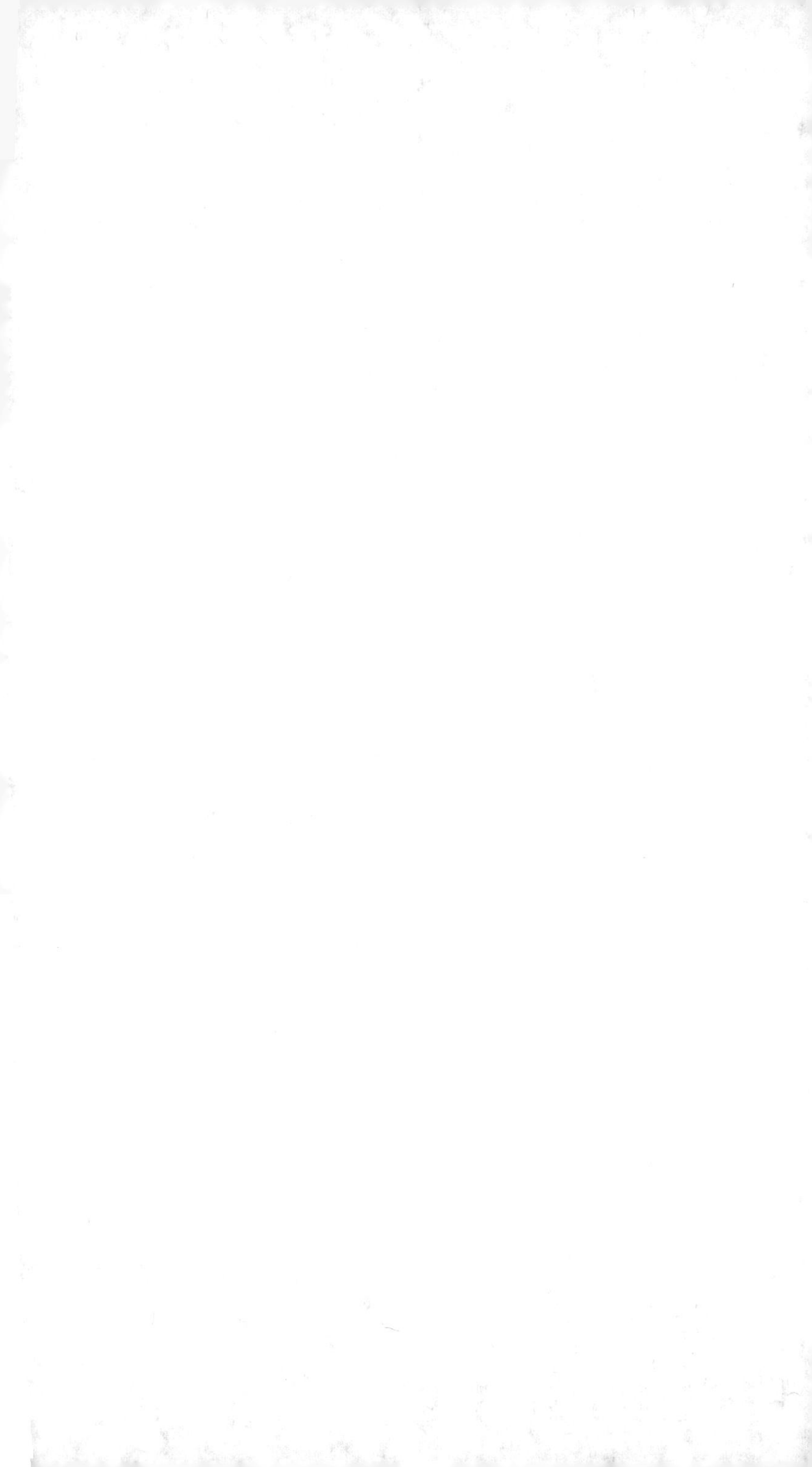